The Management of Sexuality in Residential Treatment

The Management of Sexuality in Residential Treatment

Gordon Northrup, MD
Editor

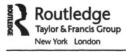

Routledge
Taylor & Francis Group
New York   London

Routledge is an imprint of the
Taylor & Francis Group, an informa business

The Management of Sexuality in Residential Treatment has also been published as *Residential Treatment for Children & Youth,* Volume 11, Number 2 1993.

Reprinted 2009 by Routledge

Library of Congress Cataloging-in-Publication Data

The Management of sexuality in residential treatment / Gordon Northrup, editor.
    p. cm.
    Includes bibliographical references and index.
    ISBN 1-56024-483-6 (acid-free-paper)
    1. Child psychotherapy–Residential treatment. 2. Adolescent psychotherapy–Residential treatment. 3. Sexually abused children–Rehabilitation. 4. Sexually abused teenagers–Rehabilitation. 5. Teenage sex offenders–Rehabilitation. 6. Children–Sexual behavior. 7. Teenagers–Sexual behavior. I. Northrup, Gordon.
RJ504.5.M355 1993
618.92' 8914–dc20

                           93-41273
                             CIP

The Management of Sexuality in Residential Treatment

CONTENTS

ABOUT THE EDITOR

Gordon Northrup, MD, is a child psychiatrist in the private practice of consultation to residential treatment schools for emotionally disturbed children and youth. A Clinical Associate at the Austin Riggs Center, he is also on the staff of the Berkshire Mental Health Center and was for many years Director of a former AAPSC child guidance clinic. Dr. Northrup has published a variety of professional papers and was Editor of *Milieu Therapy* for several years. Currently, he is Editor of the journal *Residential Treatment for Children & Youth*.

ABOUT THE CONTRIBUTORS

Robert B. Bloom, PhD, is Executive Director of the Jewish Children's Bureau in Chicago.

Richard Burnett, MSSW, ACSW, LSCSW, is Vice President for Clinical Service at The Saint Francis Academy, Incorporated, Post Office Box 1340, Salina, KS 67402, a system of nonprofit psychiatric treatment programs in Kansas, New York, and Mississippi serving youth ages ten to eighteen.

Grant Charles, MSW, RSW, is an instructor in the Child and Youth Care Programme at Lethbridge College in Lethbridge, Alberta, Canada.

Heather Coleman, MSW, is Assistant Professor in the Faculty of Social Work at the University of Calgary (Lethbridge Division) in Lethbridge, Alberta, Canada.

Alan Keith-Lucas, PhD, first received an MA in English at Cambridge, and then went on to receive an MS in Social Administration at Western Reserve and a PhD in Political Science from Duke. He is the author of 16 books, among them *Giving and Taking Help* and *Group Child Care as a Family Service,* 150 articles, chapters, and the like. He is now Alumni Distinguished Professor Emeritus at the University of North Carolina and is the Book Department Editor for *Residential Treatment for Children & Youth.*

Jane Matheson, MSW, RSW, is Director of Residential Treatment at Woods Homes in Calgary, Alberta, Canada.

Danilo E. Ponce, MD, is Professor of Child and Adolescent Psychiatry in the Department of Psychiatry at the University of Hawaii,

John A. Burns School of Medicine. He is particularly interested in the clinical applications of developmental theory; Eastern wisdom traditions (e.g., Buddhism, Taoism, Sufism, and Vedanta), and western psychotherapy; and counter-transference issues in the youth services field.

Douglas Powers, MD, is Child-Adolescent Psychiatrist and Distinguished Professor in the College of Education and Allied Professions, The University of North Carolina at Charlotte. He was formerly the Book Review Editor of *Residential Treatment for Children & Youth.*

Cheryl Rathbun, MSW, LSCSW, is Social Work Supervisor at Saint Francis at Ellsworth, Post Office Box 127, Ellsworth KS 67439, one of Saint Francis Academy's related corporations.

Raymond Schimmer, MA, is currently Assistant Executive Director for Residence and Education at the Parsons Child and Family Center in Albany, NY. He worked previously at the Tufts-New England Medical Center's psychiatric day hospital for children in Boston, MA, and at the Walker School, in Needham, MA. Mr. Schimmer received a BA from Hunter College, and an MAT from the Harvard Graduate School of Education.

Seran E. Schug, MCAT, is a Movement Psychotherapist at Mathom House in Bucks County, PA, a residential treatment facility for adolescent sex offenders, where she provides individual and group therapy to residents utilizing and integrating psychodynamic, cognitive-behavioral, and creative arts approaches to treatment. Prior to this appointment, Ms. Schug was Movement Therapist at The Devereux Foundation, Devon, PA. She has presented her work at national conferences and currently serves as adjunct faculty member in the Creative Arts in Therapy Department of Hahneman University. Seran also works as a consultant to organizations interested in the psychotherapeutic use of the arts and is currently engaged in a project at the Doylestown Center for Psychological Services.

Bruce S. Zahn, MA, is Director of Psychological Services and Cognitive Therapy Programs at Presbyterian Medical Center of Philadelphia, PA. Mr. Zahn has extensive experience in residential treatment and has recently collaborated with David D. Burns, MD, author of *The Feeling Good Handbook*, to adapt cognitive therapy to inpatient and residential psychiatric programs. Prior to his appointment at Presbyterian, Mr. Zahn was Senior Psychologist at The Devereux Foundation in Devon, PA. Mr. Zahn is a doctoral candidate in psychology at Temple University, and maintains an active private practice in clinical psychology.

Foreword

The word "love" is discordant, even shocking, when coupled with articles on the practical management of sexuality. Nevertheless, I have placed *Children and Love* first because the personal relationship between staff and the youngster being treated is where the trouble—and the good—starts. The residential treatment of youngsters includes socialization and parenting as well as psychotherapy; it therefore must include elements of loving, and especially for a direct care worker, direct body contact, as well as candid appreciation of the youngster's gender social role (masculinity and femininity). Responding to these needs does not include physical sexuality, of course, but carries a grave risk of being misunderstood as that by other staff, parents, and program inspectors. The risk extends to other children viewing the interaction and even to the child concerned, especially if he or she has been sexually abused.

Staff Reactions to Young People Who Have Been Sexually Abused carries on this theme: it is a careful survey of personal relationship problems of direct care staff with these youngsters, such as attack, avoidance, arousal, rescue efforts, and the like. Though the emphasis is on direct care staff, no staff is exempt, and even the whole residential treatment center may at times "replicate the dynamics of isolation and strong adherence to authority that exist in abusive homes . . . . Children in residential programs may be especially vulnerable to abuse from staff due to a combination of learned victim behavior, intense attachment needs and increased reliance and dependency on adults." The authors emphasize the staff's need for support and training in dealing with their reactions, and remedial administrative measures are presented.

[Haworth co-indexing entry note]: "Foreword." Northrup, Gordon. Co-published simultaneously in *Residential Treatment for Children & Youth* (The Haworth Press, Inc.) Vol. 11, No. 2, 1993, pp. *xxi-xxiii*; and: *The Management of Sexuality in Residential Treatment* (ed: Gordon Northrup) The Haworth Press, Inc., 1993, pp. *xvii-xix*. Multiple copies of this article/chapter may be purchased from The Haworth Document Delivery Center [1-800-3-HAWORTH; 9:00 a.m. - 5:00 p.m. (EST)].

xvii

After this general survey, two articles offer practical advice on managing everyday sexuality. *Some Medical Implications of Sexuality* . . . is not about physiology, but is in fact a humane survey of minor sex problems in the milieu: masturbation, sex play, sex talk, and the like, and how to respond to them, all introduced by a gently humorous poem in blank verse. A single such problem, *The Impact of Sexually-Stimulating Materials* . . . (such as Playboy magazine) is considered thoroughly in the following article. It includes a review of the pertinent studies, a characteristic summary being that "simple exposure to non-violent, non-degrading sexual depictions, irrespective of their explicitness, does not appear to cause increased viewer aggression or attitudinal changes in laboratory situations." Thus, the studies suggest that violence and coercion, not sexuality, are the problems; that viewing violent or degrading sexual material offers a potential for harm. This article presents notes on policy development that are developed fully in the author's article . . . *The Governance of Sexual Behavior* . . . in Volume 11, Number 1 of *Residential Treatment for Children & Youth.*

The first of two treatment programs is . . . *Treatment of Adolescent Sexual Offenders.* . . . The staff of an open center for 28 conduct-disordered boys aged 12 to 17 found that 10 of them had committed sexual offenses. The article discusses the development and course of a program including group therapy, individual counselling, sex education, journal writing, and family therapy. It documents some indications of modestly successful outcomes. Many practical points are made, for example, teaching the offender how to discuss the offense with the victim, and in family counselling "the patient should not be present with the victim until he owns the sexual offense."

The Survivors Project . . . describes an eight week program for five adolescent girls in an open residential setting, including structured process, stress skills training, and movement therapy groups, in addition to the customary psychotherapy. Treatment centers considering such a program will welcome the ample details, such as the note about the therapist's liability to "strong countertransference feelings of anger, disregard, and hurt. As co-therapists, we found it beneficial to work through these feelings outside the group sessions," because they could then more easily accept the members' anger and fear. They go on, ". . . many intense feelings were projected onto the male co-therapist, which needed to be adsorbed rather than directly confronted, because confrontation might be perceived as being too intrusive and threatening to their safety. For example, the *Conflicted Emoter* (a group member) consistently projected her fears of being looked at as a sexual object . . . and demanded, 'Stop looking at me!'," which request he respected.

The final two articles deal with the management of incidents of abuse. In summarizing the first, *When Staff Members Sexually Abuse Children in Residential Care* I cannot do better than quote the authors' precis: "When an agency staff member is accused of sexually abusing a client, administration is faced with the Solomonic tasks of balancing the necessity of protecting the child, supporting the staff, and maintaining the integrity and regulation of the agency. This article presents practical suggestions for managing the agency through such a crisis."

To return to our opening considerations, maintaining the therapeutic personal relationship while dealing with sexual issues causes great difficulty for most staff because they are dealing with their own conflicts. It is a common problem; as Freud said, sexuality most openly expresses the primitive areas of the personality. *Erotic Countertransference Issues in a Residential Treatment Center* deals directly with the issues. The presentation is neatly divided into four types: staff-induced versus patient-induced issues that are conscious versus unconscious, and these four types are discussed in detail with examples of management, varying with the degree of experience of the staff.

This whole group of articles on managing sexuality in residential treatment supplements the last issue of *Residential Treatment for Children & Youth* (Volume 11, Number 1) which was also published in hardcover as *Sexual Abuse and Residential Treatment* (The Haworth Press, Inc., 1992).

Gordon Northrup, MD
Editor

Children and Love

Alan Keith-Lucas, PhD

Most young children need a lot more physical affection and admiration than they get, even in a normal family. This is particularly true of little girls, and they need it from a man, and in a sense, just for being little girls. It is an important factor in them learning to like themselves and be glad that they are girls, especially at an age when boys tend to be stronger and have more freedom than girls. One hopes that they get it from their fathers–and being "daddy's girl" is a valued status–but not all do, and the ones we see in Children's Homes have often missed out on the experience altogether.

Even before the present concern about child sexual abuse we tended to discourage this need in little girls. Little girls were taught to be "ladylike" and not to seek attention from men. The most ladylike group of little girls I have ever seen were in a cottage that was controlled by a maiden lady who sheltered them from any outside contacts. The cottage had a fine reputation. There was never a peep out of it. I am sure the housemother did not appreciate me visiting. She and I sat on the porch as the children came back from school and without looking in my direction went indoors to change their clothes, until she made a fatal mistake. As nine-year-old Leta came up the steps she said to her, "Why don't you say hello to Dr. Keith-Lucas?"

Leta swam-dived onto my lap, nearly knocking me over. As soon

The author may be written at 705 Greenwood, Chapel Hill, NC 27514.

This article was previously published in "Encounters with Children: Stories that Help Us Understand and Help Them," North American Association of Christians in Social Work, St. Davids, PA, 1991.

[Haworth co-indexing entry note]: "Children and Love." Keith-Lucas, Alan. Co-published simultaneously in *Residential Treatment for Children & Youth* (The Haworth Press, Inc.) Vol. 11, No. 2, 1993, pp. 1-8; and: *The Management of Sexuality in Residential Treatment* (ed: Gordon Northrup) The Haworth Press, Inc., 1993, pp. 1-8. Multiple copies of this article/chapter may be purchased from The Haworth Document Delivery Center [1-800-3-HAWORTH; 9:00 a.m. - 5:00 p.m. (EST)].

as she was settled she told me "Don't you sit under the apple trees with any one else but me" (a popular song at the time). The other girls poured out on the porch and fought and bit to dispossess Leta and take her place. After I'd gone the housemother paddled each one of the girls, which made me very sad but it was this incident that persuaded the administration to put in family cottages with a housefather in each. They also employed a "tame grandfather," a retired widower who did odd jobs around the campus and also always had a hug for a little girl, or a boy for that matter.

Since the discovery of the extent of child sexual abuse, men in children's homes have had to be very careful. Almost any physical contact can be interpreted as abuse. Even fathers are suspect. An eight-year-old who likes to join her parents for breakfast in bed on Sundays is told always to get in on her mother's side. A woman teacher who used to pat children on their backs when they had done something well now tells them to go pat themselves. This is tragic. Children, it's true, must be protected from unwelcomed attention, but not at the cost of denying them one of their deepest needs.

We sometimes forget, I think, how desolate some children can be.

Wanda, a seven-year-old, was one of the saddest children I ever met. She was either crying, had just stopped crying or was getting ready to cry. On the last day of my visit I realised that I could not leave without saying goodbye to her, so I went to her cottage. Wanda clung to me with what I described later in a poem as a 'tetanic clutch.' "Don't leave me," she sobbed.

I told Wanda I had to go, but would not forget her, and would be back next year. "No, you won't," she said. "You'll die during the year. That's what always happens to people who love me."

The Home did a beautiful job with Wanda. Wanda was by then in a group home. They brought her to the main campus to meet me as soon as I arrived next year. Wanda came in smiling. "Wanda, I did come back," I said. "You know," she said, "I was just beginning to believe that you would."

It was, I think, rather pathetic that Wanda should see me, who had only known her for two or three days, as a person who loved her. I had paid her some attention because she was so miserable. She wasn't an attractive child whom people like to pet. In fact to most people she was a sniveling little brat. I am blessed, the Lord knows why, with a great deal of affection for the Wandas of this world, the scraps of humanity with enormous burdens to bear. Wanda had seen her father kill her mother and had been threatened with death if she ever told, and a beloved grandmother had died shortly afterwards.

I make this point because it is important that one really does love a child, not merely apply love as a poultice. A child recently asked me a question I had never been asked before.

Emma, eight, diagnosed as schizophrenic, one of two girls along with six boys in a group home in England, attached herself to me almost as soon as I arrived. The other children all seemed to have some activity, but Emma didn't. Chattering mostly about her fears, it wasn't long before she found herself on my knee. I petted her a little, stroked her hair. A staff member passed. "I see Emma's found herself a boy-friend," she said. Emma turned to face me. "Do you," she said, "really *like* being kind to me?" I was glad to be able to reply, "My dear, I love it."

I could see Emma being told as part of her therapy that the staff loved her but doubting if they really meant it. Words often don't mean much to a child, when actions and body language do. Emma, a staff member told me, was more relaxed and less fearful that night than she had been any time in the Home. She needed therapy, yes, but she also needed cuddling.

Holding a child on one's knee is often the best specifically in times of stress or sadness. Patty, whose problem I'll discuss later, wanted only to be "held tight" while she waited for her mother. Betsy, five, banished to her room, not as a punishment, but because adults needed to be able to talk without her constant interruption, posted a notice on her door. What it said was, "I would like a kiss and some lap-time." And I don't think I'll ever forget the ten-year-old in my Sunday School class who asked me, as the class was dismissed, "Could I stay five minutes longer, and would you let me sit on your knee? I quarreled with my sister this morning and I am feeling bad about it." These children didn't need good advice at the moment. Celia, I knew, would find a way of making it up with her sister. What she needed was affirmation. She didn't even need the whole five minutes. After I'd held her for perhaps three, she sighed, climbed down and said, "Thank you. I feel much better now."

Unloved children can be quite jealous of attention shown to others. On my visit once to a Home where I knew the children quite well, I was to meet, by arrangement, with four twelve year olds, who had asked for a private session, because, as they said, they had something to tell me. The child care worker had said, "I think I know what they want, but they'd better get it off their chests." I expected early teen-age gripes but no, as one girl explained, they thought I was neglecting them. When I came to the cottage I let the eights and nines sit on my knee. Now that they had me without the younger ones would I give them five minutes apiece? I did, but when we rejoined the others I found the younger children in tears. They felt that I had neglected them.

Yet I have known children to be generous in this respect. Years ago, in England, I used to visit a Children's Home where a dozen school-age children were left to themselves from tea-time onwards while the inadequate staff put to bed a small raft of younger ones. The four oldest, eleven year olds, two boys and two girls, stayed up the longest and became my special friends. At their insistence I'd stay until I had tucked them up in bed, as many as three nights a week. Otherwise they simply took themselves off to bed. They needed a great deal of affection. From time to time they were joined by a new child, sent from a London hospital to recuperate in the country, but the four were permanent residents.

One night Anne met me at the door. "I'm glad you came tonight," she said, "but Grace and I aren't going to sit on your knee." My first thought was that someone had told them they were too old to do so or that they themselves had become self-conscious. But Anne explained, "It isn't that we don't want to. We want to very much. But we've a new girl tonight and she is very sad. We want her to have you all by herself." The new girl was indeed sad, a child dancer and acrobat—she could tie herself into incredible knots—but so starved and neglected that her stomach was distended and every inch of her body covered with scabies, ten years old, but I would have thought her six, reeking of urine, with nits in her hair, which Anne and I combed for her and not so much sitting as lying on my lap. But when I kissed her good night, after tucking her in, she said almost the first words I had heard her say. "Thank you," she said, "for the loveliest evening I've ever had in my life."

Twelve-year-olds, such as the ones who hi-jacked me, and Anne and Grace, when they reached that age, may seem too old to sit on a man's knee. It is easy to suspect that they may have some sort of sexual motive. When met with demands to be held by children as old as eleven or twelve I used to rationalize by saying that children away from home had missed this experience at a more appropriate age, and if they didn't get it now they would still be wanting physical affection from a man at sixteen or seventeen. I saw a twelve-year-old in a Children's Home as three or four years retarded in her emotional growth. But lately one or two experiences with children who live at home has made me believe that quite a number of little girls need this kind of reassurance at an older age than I had thought. Their motives are not so much sexual as gender-related. They need appreciation from a man for being a girl. And love is often best conveyed by physical contact, by hugging and holding tight, although sometimes it is conveyed in other ways. A little black girl, the granddaughter of the woman who did our house-cleaning for us, once told me, "Oh, I am so glad to be able to talk to a man. Granny's making me a lavender dress. Do you think it would go with my complexion?" It seemed a strange question for her to ask a white man but as she said, if she asked any of the men at home they would laugh at her for being vain, and she really did want to know.

Being a girl is sometimes difficult. Nita, ten, was always beautifully dressed and would wear a dress when others were in jeans. I remarked on this to her housefather. "Yes," he said, "we want Nita to be proud of being a girl. She was the only girl in a household of seven men and boys. Even her brothers had intercourse with her nearly every night. So my wife and I bought her pretty feminine clothes. At first she wouldn't wear them, but now models them for me. I tell her how pretty she looks in them."

The housefather was helping Nita come to terms with what had happened to her just as much as if he had her in therapy in a program for sexually abused children. And it was significant that it was for him and not for his wife that she modeled her pretty things. She had now come to the point of saying, "My father did love me, but he took the wrong way of showing it." Nita avoided one reaction to having been abused sexually. She didn't become aggressively masculine or make herself deliberately unattractive. Children remember those who have been genuinely fond of them. "Poor old Lessie"–no one called her anything else–was an ungainly apparently mildly retarded child, with horrible blackened teeth when I first knew her when she was ten. I saw her again when she was twelve, which I will relate later, but then not again until she was seventeen. She met me saying, "I'm no longer the 'poor old Lessie' you used to let sit on your knee. I've even got an admirer." She was now not unattractive and the Home had fixed her teeth. I said that must make her happy, and she said yes, but ten minutes later when I was sitting in the living room, Lessie said to me, "Would you mind if just for a minute I sat on your knee again. Just for old times' sake."

In another Home I also visited after a lapse of five years, I was asked to speak in Chapel to more than three hundred children. (Homes at that time were much larger and many children stayed in them for five years or more.) In my remarks I made the rather silly comment that there were little bits of my ridiculously sentimental heart buried on the campus. For me it was full of the ghosts of long grownup children. When the children filed out two teen-agers remained. "We're Flossie and Barbara," they said. "You meant us, didn't you?" And they were right. They were the two I remembered best. Flossie at ten had written me a note thanking me for treating her "just as if I was your own little girl" and Barbara had come to me in floods of tears, just as the bell had rung for the march to the dining hall having caught her dress on a nail and torn it from her shoulder down to her waist. Luckily in those days men wore tie-pins, and I sacrificed mine to repair the damage temporarily. She said I saved her from a sure spanking.

I was addressing a meeting of social workers from both public and private agencies. Often when I make a speech I watch two or three people in the audience to gauge their reactions to what I am saying. This time my attention centered on a dark-haired young woman in the front row, whose face was vaguely familiar. Her expression was one of puzzlement.

After the session she approached me. "Do you remember me?" she asked. "You wouldn't be Janice, would you?" I said, praying that I would be right.

"Yes," she said, "I'm the one you made a special visit to when I was in the infirmary because you missed me in the cottage, and I had rheumatic fever. And reassured me I wouldn't be a cripple for life. I was ten, I think, at that time, and now I find that you are some sort of child welfare expert. So either you have changed since I knew you or one part of you is phony. You can't be both the grandfather who let us sit on your knee and told us Uncle Remus stories and didn't wear polished black shoes and at the same time be a child welfare expert. Which is the real you?"

I'm not sure that I ever convinced her that I might possibly be both. Shades of Emma and "Do you really like being kind to me?" But children know if you really love them. A child gave me a comeuppance once:

It was a huge impersonal orphanage. There were some forty or fifty little girls between the ages of six and nine, but Kim caught my attention at once. She was a beautiful child who seemed to be dying on the vine. I asked to see her case-record. Her father had killed himself the night Kim's mother died of cancer. No one had told Kim that her father was dead. She was waiting for a visit that never came. The Home did not allow its children to be adopted.

In my discussion with the staff I used Kim's case to try to help them see what they were doing to children but I decided, rather against my inclination, not to give Kim any special attention in my informal contacts with the children. When telling them stories I never sat next to Kim, or chose her as an actor. I never had her sit on my knee. I didn't want to single her out in any way and thought I had managed not to do so.

On my last day at the Home Kim presented me with her school picture. "I think you are going to need this," she said.

One result of my consultation. The Home told Kim of her father's death and found her an adoptive home.

And finally a story that seems to be too good to be true, but does make a very important point. It was told me by a child care worker.

Loma, seven, got out of bed on the wrong side that morning. She disliked everyone and every thing she saw. Since it was summer and a fine day the housemother said, in exasperation, "Why don't you go outside and see if you can't find some love. You are certainly not finding it here."

Sometime later the housemother happened to look out of the window. Lorna, with her eyes fixed on the ground, was walking up and down the lawn, covering every square foot of it. Eventually she had covered it all and came back into the house.

"Well," said the housemother, "did you find any love out there?"

"No," said Lorna. "The trouble is I don't know what love looks like."

Staff Reactions to Young People Who Have Been Sexually Abused

Grant Charles, MSW
Heather Coleman, MSW
Jane Matheson, MSW

SUMMARY. A great deal has been written in recent years about the impact and treatment of child sexual abuse. However, despite the large number of previously abused young people who reside in residential programmes, little has been written regarding intrapersonal reactions of the staff who work with these children. This article examines the various reactions found among residential workers towards young people in their care who have been sexually abused.

A tremendous amount of investigation has been conducted in the area of child sexual abuse over the past decade. Much of the work has involved determining the extent of the problem, recognizing the various indicators of possible abuse, establishing the short and long-term consequences of various types of abuse and developing of specific interventions. Despite this, relatively little study has been done developing treatment for child sexual abuse survivors who reside in residential treatment centers. This is perhaps the result of an assumption that treatment interventions developed in outpatient settings for adult survivors or child victims can be easily

---

The authors may be written at Lethbridge Community College, Lethbridge, Alberta, Canada, T1K 1L6.

[Haworth co-indexing entry note]: "Staff Reactions to Young People Who Have Been Sexually Abused." Charles, Grant, Heather Coleman, and Jane Matheson. Co-published simultaneously in *Residential Treatment for Children & Youth* (The Haworth Press, Inc.) Vol. 11, No. 2, 1993, pp. 9-21; and: *The Management of Sexuality in Residential Treatment* (ed: Gordon Northrup) The Haworth Press, Inc., 1993, pp. 9-21. Multiple copies of this article/chapter may be purchased from The Haworth Document Delivery Center [1-800-3-HAWORTH; 9:00 a.m. - 5:00 p.m. (EST)].

adapted to meet the needs of young people who are inpatients in institutions. Given the often unique needs of these young people in addition to the distinct characteristics of residential programs these assumptions may not be well founded. The work that has been conducted in regard to young people in residential programs has tended to focus upon interventions by clinicians. As such the emphasis has been upon family or individual traditional therapies. Little has been written about the dynamics of interventions by front-line child and youth care workers with abuse survivors within the residential milieu. This is surprising, given the growing evidence that many young people who reside in residential treatment centers have a history of sexual abuse (Giarretto, 1982).

Residential treatment, by its very nature, is a powerful intervention modality. The opportunity to affect positive change is quite strong given the possible range of interventions and the opportunity for intensive, growth oriented staff-young person relationships. While it is important to recognize the opportunity for positive interactions within residential settings, it is also essential to be aware of the potential for non-therapeutic interplay between the staff and the young people in their programmes who have been abused. This paper will outline several of these potential negative or non-therapeutic interactions as well as some potential preventive measures that can be taken to decrease the likelihood of their occurrence.

The dynamics of sexual abuse are pervasive, powerful and intrusive. Young people will often seek to recreate in the cottage setting the dynamics that existed in their families. This is not because they are seeking further pain but rather because they are often recreating the only experiences they have ever known. The result is a possible manifestation of abusive or dysfunctional adult-child interactions. Additionally, some workers also bring to the cottage personal unresolved issues and/or dysfunctional behaviors.

The intensity of the work that the staff are expected to perform and the severity of the symptoms of some young people whom they are in contact with can create strong reactive feelings. These feelings are often manifested through reactions of attack, avoidance, or arousal. Each of these types of reactions are counterproductive and possibly harmful to the young people in care if not dealt with immediately and appropriately (Courtois, 1988).

There are a variety of reactions that staff can experience while working with young people in residential treatment centres. Given the troubled and troubling behaviours many young people bring to the centres, it is not surprising that these reactions can be discomforting, confusing, painful and potentially harmful both to the staff and the young person. Knowledge of the reactions is therefore important for the well-being of the staff and the people in their care.

Staff who work with young people who have been sexually abused need to be fully supported in their work. Child and youth care workers also need a variety of skills when working with abuse survivors. Workers also need specialized training that considers the unique issues of working with children who have been oppressed and exploited.

Staff should be equipped with a working knowledge of the dynamics of sexual abuse. They require training that includes the identification of indicators and symptoms as well as treatment modalities, prevention issues and potential self and peer reactions to the manifestation of symptoms. Staff also need specific training regarding issues of sexuality (Lynch et al., 1990; McFadden, 1989).

Staff need to have a thorough working knowledge of the dynamics of sexual abuse to understand the potential range of interactions that can take place between themselves and the children in their care. They also need to have an understanding of the possible feelings, fears and fantasies that they could possibly experience during their work with sexually abused young people. Without such an understanding, staff could engage in destructive thought patterns, interactions or behaviours.

Without an accurate understanding of some behavioural and interactional manifestations of abuse, some staff may actually begin to blame the survivor for the victimization. This can happen when staff begin to judge the young person as malevolent and deserving of previous traumatization. For example, some survivors will act in manipulative and evasive ways so as to try to get their needs met. While these actions are dysfunctional in non-abusive settings they are basic survival skills when one is being victimized. Unless this is understood, the staff, after initially reaching out to the young person, may eventually perceive these behaviours as a rejection of them as professionals and people. This can elicit feelings of anger and hurt, culminating in the eventual rejection of the child. Once this happens it is then possible to label the young person as "unworkable." The staff can then distort this belief into a perception that the young person is bad and if so then the hurt the child has experienced in the past is in some ways justifiable (Browne, 1991; Leehan & Wilson, 1985).

The dynamic behind this distortion rests upon the belief that if one is a caring professional yet is rejected by a young person, the rejection stems from an inherent weakness or badness in the child. Coupled with this is a belief held by many people in our society that individuals who are bad should be punished and are deserving of any trauma they experience or that those who have been hurt must have been bad or else they would not have been hurt. This also allows individuals to dissociate from any sense of societal responsibility for the victimization (Bagley & King, 1990). Therapist impotence becomes readily translated into that of the "unworkable client" (Reynolds-Meija & Levitan, 1990).

It is important for staff to be aware of the context in which behaviours were learned. It is also important to recognize that dysfunctional behaviours are an integral component of the personality and as such will not immediately disappear because of an expression of caring. Without this awareness the staff may personalize their experiences with abuse survivors rather than acknowledge that the behaviors of the young person are manifestations of reactions to abuse.

There also can be a tendency for staff unconsciously to reject or avoid some abuse survivors because of the tremendous psychological and emotional demands the young people may place upon the child and youth care workers. The pain many survivors manifest can be overwhelming to people around them, resulting in rejection of the young person. Many survivors also need to test constantly the limits of relationships to ensure that the adults will behave as they say they will and that the relationship will remain non-exploitive. All these behaviours are difficult to deal with even with knowledge of the dynamics of victimization. They are nearly impossible to deal with if one does not have an understanding of their origins (Browne, 1991; Leehan & Wilson, 1985).

The enormity of the pain and the seemingly pervasive extent of damage to some survivors of sexual abuse can provoke for some staff a sense of inadequacy and helplessness. Staff members may collude with the victim's denial of abuse (Reynolds-Mejia & Levitan, 1990). They may begin to think that they have inadequate training for the task of facilitating the healing of the young person. They also focus upon the apparent lack of resources within the community and the agency to deal with abuse with the consequence that they begin to develop an attitude of helplessness. Others may react with disgust at the details of the abuse and feel unable to connect with the survivor. Still other staff may experience guilt about not being able to undo the pain the young person has experienced. Ultimately, the result of each of these possible reactions may be the unconscious rejection of the young person who will internalize the rejection not as a staff issue but as the extension of her own non-worth (Catherall, 1991; Courtois, 1988; McElroy & McElroy, 1991).

Furthermore, some staff have themselves been victims of sexual abuse. This can create some potentially complex dynamics if they have not dealt with their own victimization. The staff member may not be able to listen to the child discuss their abuse without reliving her own experience. This can result in the expression of previously repressed and painful memories, causing the worker to avoid interactions with the young person, which in turn reinforces the young person's belief that she is not worthy of other people's care or positive attention (Herman, 1981; Porter, 1984).

Rejection of the young person also can occur because the knowledge of the child's situation can cause a staff member who has never experienced abuse to begin to feel vulnerable. The knowledge that such victimization occurs can shatter a worker's sense of safety and innocence (Reynolds-Mejia & Levitan, 1990). This is a form of contact abuse or secondary victimization whereby the worker experiences a destruction of her world view as a safe and secure place. The staff member can also feel vulnerable because of a primitive fear of becoming contaminated through exposure to a "damaged" person. These reactions, though not based on a logical response, are real to the worker (Bagley & King, 1990; Courtois, 1988).

Another potential consequence of a staff member's unresolved victimization can be an expression of rage toward the parents of the young person. In this scenario, the worker does not permit the child to express feelings; rather the worker attempts to express feelings on behalf of the child (Reynolds-Mejia & Levitan, 1990). The anger may be directed toward the offending person for hurting the child or the non-offending parent for apparently not protecting the young person. While these feelings are understandable, the staff member may ultimately express emotions that the child does not yet share, thereby evoking defensive reactions in the child. It can also create loyalty confusions for the young person between the staff member and the parents. It is probable that the worker will be rejected by the child in this process thus negating the possible impact of any future positive interactions (Catherall, 1991; Herman, 1981).

Another possible staff-young person interaction is the over-identification by the worker with the survivor where the worker mistakes sympathy for empathy (Reynolds-Mejia & Levitan, 1990). Rather than rejecting the individual, the staff member becomes the strong caring parent the child never experienced. This "good parent" often overprotects the young person and can inhibit the expected transference of hurt and anger that most survivors need to direct toward an adult with whom they feel a sense of safety. The transference process is a critical step in healing that may not happen if the worker-child relationship turns into a pseudo-parent-child relationship. This tendency to compete with the parents of abuse victims threatens survivors' self-esteem and ultimately discounts the parents as important people in the child's life (Reynolds-Mejia & Levitan, 1990). Victims have been taught to suppress strong feelings around parents. The young person may, in this type of relationship, do what she perceives the worker wants her to do rather than what is in her best interests thus recreating similar dynamics to the previous abusive relationships. Staff therefore need to master their tendencies to over-identify with victims (Haaken & Schlaps, 1991; Herman, 1981).

Such rescue behaviour can also be manifested in a desire to ensure that the young person never again experiences pain. The child's existing strength is ignored in the process and rather than being accepted as a person who has experienced trauma, is treated as a fragile doll who must be protected from past horrors. Sometimes the survivor is romanticized as a heroine who has survived a battle with the evil forces of the world. The result is a further dehumanization of the young person (Courtois, 1988).

This attitude toward survivors can become quite confusing when workers encounter dealing with young people who have been victimized who are now abusing or who are suspected of abusing other children. As the evidence increases that some victims, especially but not exclusively males, in turn victimize others, workers are confronted with a dilemma. For "romanticized" survivors, the worker may ignore or minimize the indicators that the individual is abusing other people. This has negative consequences not just for the new victim but also for the offender. Another possibility is that staff will become quite angry or enraged when confronted with evidence that their romanticized survivor is hurting other people. Their impression of the young person can change from that of an all good victim to an all bad offender. This is as dehumanizing and non-therapeutic as treating the individual as a heroine.

Perhaps the most disturbing reactions that the staff can experience have to do with issues regarding sexuality. These feelings can be uncomfortable because of the expectation that adults should not harbour sexual feelings toward young people and also because of the expectation that workers must always maintain clear boundaries between themselves and their clients. Part of the discomfort also arises from the taboo in parts of society in discussing sexuality. Survivor treatment forces workers to address directly these issues (Briere, 1989; Gillman & Whitlock, 1989; Porter, 1984).

Some workers may become aroused by the details of the abuse and by exposure to someone who has been sexually "damaged." This morbid fascination with the knowledge of forbidden activities can create a form of privileged voyeurism, stimulating sexual fantasies. This can be discomforting for staff who may be so disconcerted by their feelings that they will repress or refuse to admit the existence of the arousal state. The worker may then begin to avoid the young person or the topic of abuse as a means of denying the feelings. Occasionally the worker may fixate on the details of the abuse and experience a vicarious arousal at the expense of the survivor (Courtois, 1988; Porter, 1984).

Staff also need to be aware of the tendency of some survivors to sexualize all of their relationships. The victim has been taught by the offender that she is only important insofar as she sexually satisfies adults. This socialization can be carried into relationships with other adults and the young person may display seductive behaviors as means of sexualizing the relationship. This creates much discomfort for workers who may in turn respond by avoiding the child rather than addressing the inappropriateness of the behavior. By not confronting the young person with the behavior, the worker may be providing a powerful tool to use against him or her. The worker, through his or her silence, may also be inadvertently condoning the behavior (McElroy & McElroy, 1991; Porter, 1984).

The sexualized behavior of the young person potentially places the child at risk of further abuse by staff members who are exploitive or who have their own boundary issues. Given the power imbalances that exist in many centers between staff and young people, it would not be difficult for some staff to be able to use their positions of authority to sexually exploit a young person. The possibility exists that the survivor's learned helplessness responses coupled with her sexualized behavior will be seen by some staff as a form of permission to engage in exploitive sexual behavior. This is, of course, a distortion of reality which will create further harm for the child (Bagley & King, 1990).

Perhaps most importantly, workers need assistance in developing a calm, non-judgmental attitude toward working with survivors. Staff members need training in being able to respond to young people who are manifesting victim symptomatology in such a manner that the necessary boundaries and limits are established and maintained. They also need to be able not to personalize the child's projections of anger or sexualization (Crenshaw, 1988).

Workers may also require assistance in reconceptualizing and changing many traditional ways they interact with young people. Some staff must be taught that it is critical for them to respect the privacy and bodies of the young people with whom they are working. Touching games such as tickling or wrestling or sitting on the edge of a child's bed may be interpreted by a young person as a prelude to abuse rather than nurturing activities. People who have been abused cannot always differentiate between sexual and nurturing touch. Staff should recognize that no one should touch another without permission. This applies to staff-child as well as staff-staff interactions.

Staff also need to receive an appropriate level of supervision and support. They need the opportunity to develop new skills and knowledge in addition to the opportunity to integrate these skills into practice. Supervision is critical in this process, particularly for the exploration of attitudes and reactions that may impede effective work with survivors of abuse.

Many previously mentioned issues are difficult for workers to discuss. Despite this, workers need to be encouraged to discuss not only with their supervisors but also with their peers the various reactions they may be experiencing. This encouragement is particularly important regarding any of the issues related to sexuality. The perceived forbidden topics of discussion are probably the ones that are making the workers most uncomfortable and are therefore the ones that need the most supportive supervisory attention (Crenshaw, 1988; Herman, 1981).

It must also be recognized that the high incidence of unreported abuse in the general adult population means that a significant proportion of staff members in an agency will themselves have been abused (Porter, 1984). These individuals need support to begin to deal with their own traumatization. The agency must recognize that some of these individuals may have quite strong reactions as they are exposed to the pain of the young person. These reactions need to be supported rather than censured with the ultimate goal being to help them work through their own pain. This is not to say that the agency is responsible for the treatment of its own staff but rather that it is responsible to support workers who experience trauma as, in part, a consequence of their work.

Workers who are neither provided with specialized training nor appropriate support and supervision will not be effective or persevering. They may be detrimental in their interactions with young people who have been sexually abused. Agencies have a responsibility to ensure that this does not happen by creating a work culture that is supportive to the professional and personal growth of staff members and ultimately the young people in their care.

Child sexual abuse is a pervasive problem within the community. The values and belief systems which support its presence in the general society also exist within helping agencies. In fact, residential centers at times replicate the dynamics of isolation and strong adherence to authority that exist in abusive families. As such, it should never be assumed that abuse does not happen in residential treatment centers. Indeed children in residential programmes may be especially vulnerable to abuse from staff due to a combination of learned victim behavior, intense attachment needs and increased reliance and dependency on adults (Rogers, 1988, Siskind, 1987).

Information on the extent of sexual abuse within residential centers is sparse (Groze, 1990; Bloom, 1992). Bloom (1992) suggests that abuse in residential centers may occur at twice the rate that abuse occurs in families. This is due, in part, to the secretive nature of abuse relationships and the hesitation of victims to report abuse. However, it is also due to the tendency of staff not to report suspected abuse unless the evidence is blatant (Rindfleisch & Bean, 1988). There also is an apparent tendency for people to overlook the possible indicators of abuse because they believe that it should not occur in a supposed caring environment. What should not be there cannot be there (Nunno & Motz, 1988). There may also be a tendency for agencies and government licensing bodies to minimize the extent of the problem for political reasons since if in-depth investigations and monitoring did occur it might uncover more cases than the system could handle (Rindfleisch & Bean, 1988; Rindfleisch & Hicho, 1987). However, recent information gathered from adult survivors who were in treatment for childhood incest reveals that up to thirty percent of them have been sexually exploited by members of the helping professions (Armsworth, 1989). While this figure is not conclusive it does suggest that professional ethics are not necessarily a deterrent to the abuse of clients.

It would appear that the young people who are at highest risk for abuse or reabuse are those who are the most isolated from the community. Young people who are newly admitted to a programme, who have been in prior out-of-home placements and who have little or no family contact appear to be particularly susceptible to exploitation by staff (Siskind, 1987). The young people who are the most vulnerable, needy and dependent are the very ones most likely to be abused.

Workers who abuse children in their care do so for a variety of reasons. Some are clearly paedophiles who seek employment in residential centers so as to have easy access to vulnerable children. However, it appears that the most likely type of abuse within residential programmes is single episode assault of a non-penetrative nature perpetuated by a worker lacking in emotional maturity. These individuals have poor impulse control and lack clear boundaries between themselves and the people in their care. When these people come into the type of close and intense contact with vulnerable youth as often happens in residential settings they may confuse their own need for love and acceptance with the needs of the young person (Moriarty, 1990; Siskind, 1987).

Abuse is most likely to happen in settings where there is minimal staff supervision and support. Agencies within which the staff feel disempowered or maltreated by senior administration or that have poorly developed hiring procedures tend to higher suspected rates of abuse. People who do not have a strong sense of professional identity also seem more likely to cross interactional boundaries (Moriarty, 1990; McFadden, 1989; Siskind, 1987).

The solution to the problem is relatively straightforward. Allegations by children in care should be taken seriously and the first step is the protection of children. If the perpetrator is well-liked, the child may be scapegoated by other residential staff (Bloom, 1992). Staff need support and supervision within the workplace. Agencies need to attempt to reduce the powerlessness, isolation, and stresses the workers can feel within the treatment center. Support has to be given to workers to deal with their own personal issues before these issues are played out on the young people in the programmes. Workers also need to be supported in the recognition of the importance of their work. The development of a sense of professional identity with clear role expectations needs to be encouraged (Durkin, 1981; McFadden, 1987; Moriarty, 1990).

Agencies also have to develop clear and comprehensive hiring polices and practices that discourage the employment of sexually exploitive or socially immature individuals. The latter group of people can often be identified through a rigorous structured interview process that seeks to determine the overall competency and personality characteristics of the applicant. However, this process is unlikely to identify the paedophile because their personality characteristics may be similar to those of an "ideal" staff member (Moriarty, 1990). They tend to present as good listeners who tend to have quite positive, almost idealized, attitudes toward children. Many such individuals will not appear on criminal record checks because few paedophiles are ever charged with criminal offenses.

Child sexual abuse is a pervasive problem in our society. The damage done to childhood victims is often severe and long-lasting. The children who are the most traumatized often end up in residential programmes because of the severity of their symptoms. Centers have the potential to offer these young people powerful assistance in the healing process. Unfortunately, the centers can also be the sites of further exploitation and harm. The direction toward health or harm depends upon the quality of the staff and the culture of the agency.

REFERENCES

Arnsworth, M. W. (1989). Therapy of incest survivors: Abuse or support. *Child Abuse and Neglect, 13,* 549-562.

Bagley, C., & King, K. (1990). *Child sexual abuse: The search for healing.* London: Tavistock/Routledge.

Bloom, R. (1992). When staff members sexually abuse children in residential care. *Child Welfare, LXXI*(2), 131-145.

Briere, J., Zaidi, L. Y. (1989). Sexual abuse histories and sequelae in female psychiatric emergency room patients. *American Journal of Psychiatry, 146*(12), 1602-1606.

Browne, A. (1991). The victims' experience: Pathways to disclosure. *Psychotherapy, 28*(1), 150-156.

Catherall, D. R. (1991). Aggression and projective identification in the treatment of victims. *Psychotherapy, 28*(1), 145-149.

Courtois, C. A. (1988). *Healing the incest wounds: Adult survivors in therapy.* New York: W. W. Norton & Company.

Crenshaw, D. A. (1988). Responding to sexual acting out. In C. E. Schaefer & A. J. Swanson (Eds.), *Children in residential care* (pp. 50-75). New York: Van Nostrand Reinhold.

Durkin, R. (1981). Institutional child abuse from a family systems perspective: A working paper. *Child and Youth Services,* 4(1/2), 15-22.

Giarretto, H. (1982). *Integrated treatment of child sexual abuse: A treatment and training manual.* Palo Alto: Science and Behavior Books.

Gillman R., & Whitlock, K. (1989). Sexuality: A neglected component of child sexual abuse education and training. *Child Welfare, LXVIII*(5), 317-329.

Groze, V. (1990). An exploratory investigation into institutional mistreatment. *Children and Youth Services Review, 12*, 229-241.

Haaken, J., & Schlaps, A. (1991). Incest resolution and the objectification of sexual abuse. *Psychotherapy, 28*(1), 39-47.

Herman, J. L (1981). *Father-daughter incest.* Cambridge: Harvard University Press.

Leehan, J., & Wilson, L. (1985). *Grown-up abused children.* Springfield: Charles C Thomas.

Lynch, B. F., Condon, R. H., Newell, D., & Regan, M. (1990). Positive social interaction in the treatment of male sexual abuse victims. *Residential Treatment for Children & Youth, 7*(3), 59-73.

McElroy, L P., & McElroy, R. A. (1991). Countertransference issues in the treatment of incest families. *Psychotherapy, 28*(1), 48-54.

McFadden, E. J. (1989). The sexually abused child in specialized foster care. *Child and Youth Services, 12*(1/2), 91-105.

Moriarty, A. (1990). Deterring the molester and abuser: Pre-employment testing for child and youth care workers. *Child and Youth Care Quarterly, 19*(1), 59-65.

Nunno, M. A., & Motz, J. K. (1988). The development of an effective response to the abuse of children in out-of-home care. *Child Abuse and Neglect, 12*, 521-528.

Porter, R. (1984). *Child sexual abuse within the family.* London: Tavistock Publications.

Reynolds, P. & Levitan, S. (1990). Countertransference issues in the in-home treatment of child sexual abuse. *Child Welfare, LXIX*(1), 53-61.

Rindfleisch, N., & Bean, G. J. (1988). Willingness to report abuse and neglect in residential facilities. *Child Abuse and Neglect, 12*, 15-26.

Rindfleisch, N., & Hicho, D. (1987). Institutional child protection: Issues in programme development and implementation. *Child Welfare, LXVI*(4), 329-341.

Rogers, R. (1988). *Discussion paper: An overview of issues and concerns related to the sexual abuse of children in Canada.* Ottawa: Health and Welfare Canada.

Siskind, A. B. (1987). Issues in institutional child sexual abuse: The abused, the abuser and the system. *Residential Treatment for Children & Youth, 4*(2), 9-30.

Some Medical Implications
of Sexuality in Residential Centers

THE MINI-EPIDEMIC

An epidemic raged that spring
a rash of mini-sex they said
at the children's home
the kids were loose
adults uptight

As available shaman I was called
to exorcise the evil
gathering paraphernalia
of trade I went inside
for incantations

We anatomized and philosophized
we talked of many things
they asked a thousand
questions and one
I'm sure I'll not forget

This article is reprinted from *Residential Treatment for Children & Youth*
Volume 8, Number 2, pp. 83-96, © 1990 by The Haworth Press, Inc.

The author may be written at 5517 Eagle Lake Dr. S., Charlotte, NC 28217.

[Haworth co-indexing entry note]: "Some Medical Implications of Sexuality in Residential Centers." Powers, Douglas. Co-published simultaneously in *Residential Treatment for Children & Youth* (The Haworth Press, Inc.) Vol. 11, No. 2, 1993, pp. 23-36; and: *The Management of Sexuality in Residential Treatment* (ed: Gordon Northrup) The Haworth Press, Inc., 1993, pp. 23-36. Multiple copies of this article/chapter may be purchased from The Haworth Document Delivery Center [1-800-3-HA-WORTH; 9:00 a.m. - 5:00 p.m. (EST)].

When curiosities finally lagged
one so far silent boy raised a hand
wha-wha-what's in a fa-fa-fart
he stammered while others sniggered
loud and rolled their eyes

I hesitated trying to recall
lost chemistry from away back when
dredging finally
from the depths
methane and H_2SO_4

So that epidemic spring
we dissipated evil
and explicated farts
while mini-sex recovered
or went underground
perhaps

Sexual problems among children in residence are common, and the degree of severity can and does reach alarming proportions in a population so young. Perhaps the nature and degree of such problems is not surprising when the distorted lives of the children are considered.

Whatever accounts for all the changing sexual attitudes and expressions, it is clear that more children are now being admitted into residential treatment with more florid sexual histories than have been presented in the past. There is wide-spread early sexual stimulation and experience, sexual abuse, incest, early and late pregnancies, early infections with venereal disease, and early prostitution by both boys and girls.

Medical considerations can emerge in every darkened corner. And the spectre of *AIDS* in babies, children and adolescents has produced a *dance macabre*.

Some of the more common sexual problems in residential groups of troubled children will be discussed, and where appropriate medical implications will be mentioned. The problems can create extraordinary difficulty for the children, staff, and community.

MASTURBATION

Masturbation is a common complaint about children from the line staff in residential care. Such activity may take place in living areas, school, recreation or wherever. The problem can be one of continual masturbation, but more commonly it is one of location. The child simply disregards social convention or is unaware of it and masturbates openly wherever inclined. Staff concern is not about any ill effect from the act itself but about the inappropriateness of it.

In attempting to socialize such a child, staff should be careful not to say or do anything which will further isolate the child from the significant persons around him. At times in different cultures the prevailing corrective action for an adult to take when confronted with a masturbating child was to threaten excision or mutilation of the offensive part. Supposedly this threat left the rest of that particular child well and happy thereafter. Such threats are still around, though hopefully not so commonly as formerly.

A more efficacious attitude for adults is a consistent and sustained attempt to provide gratifying human social relationships which will help move a child out of isolation and thus render the child's auto-erotic work less necessary. The act of masturbating is not condemned in itself, only the inappropriateness of the open, continual activity. Rewards, both tangible and social, are sometimes helpful to the child as motivators in decreasing the frequency and in encouraging a change of location for the activity. Auto-erotic activity as a private act is not the target of therapeutic effort unless the child is ridden by guilt and anxiety.

With a non-punitive, therapeutic attitude by staff, most children in residential treatment who have a masturbation problem are helped to control the behavior themselves. As people relationships become more important, children are more likely to honor adult expectations of them.

PROFANE SEX TALK

Sometimes parents or surrogate parents who have a troubled child in residential treatment (or group care) will return the child after a home visit declaring that their child is learning words and expressions that are unacceptable to them. They demand that the agency "do something about all those other 'bad children.'" This can reach ludicrous levels, for sometimes it is the child about whom the concern has been expressed who is known by all, children and staff alike, as one of the most "foul-speaking" children in residence.

There are troubled children in residential settings who have not been exposed to the four-letter words concentrating on certain bodily parts and functions. Most children, however, have some familiarity with the words; and some children have been reared before a steady barrage of such language.

The language, that is sometimes colorful, rhythmic and expressive on the tips of skilled tongues, can serve multiple purposes. It may be used playfully to attract the attention of other children or adults. It may be provocative and seductive; or it may be an outright proposition. It may be used as a blustery cover for fearful feelings or self-perceived weaknesses. It may be used as a deterrent if a youngster is fearful that another child will harm him. It can be a substitute for physical force if one child is afraid that in attacking another child he may injure or kill that child. In the residential setting it is often used as a method of testing adults to see just what they will tolerate and what limits they will set and what power of enforcement they have. Children on home visits may use it before their parents as a weapon directed against the residential staff, the aim being to "get staff in trouble" or "to get my parents to take me out of this damn place."

So there are many functions that vulgarity serves, from affection to rage, with mixtures of both in different strengths. The use of such language by children cannot be "stamped out" any more than it can be for adults, even though one might wish that at times.

As with masturbation, the social expectations of significant adults are important in the eventual dissipation of the undesirable language. Staff recognition of what its use means at a particular time for a particular child is important—for then that child can be helped to recognize these feelings and also be helped to find other, more socially acceptable means of expressing these feelings. Modeling after adults and admired, valued peers will become a factor in changing children's language. Parents of some children will need help in understanding their child (and themselves) in relationship to vulgar and profane language use.

Lastly, most children are probably not going to stop the use of such language completely. Most of them will, however, learn a sense of appropriateness; and as their underlying and related problems lessen, they will no longer have the need to rely on this language to so great an extent.

PARTICIPATORY SEX PLAY

Probably most young children, if they are relatively healthy, engage in some kind of participatory sex play with another child or other children at one time or another. There may be a twosome, threesome or group affair; and children may be the same sex or the opposite sex. Adults do not say much about their own early-childhood sex experiences for good reason: We repress many early memories or recall them only with difficulty under certain circumstances; we are keenly cognizant of social attitudes regarding certain sexual matters, hence we may become anxious if we do recall early sexual activity. With residual anxiety about our own early sexuality, we may tend to become alarmed at the activities of new generations.

Sexual experimentation among children in residential settings does occur and can cause much concern among staff when discovered. Concern of the staff may be partially related to what it perceives to be the disapproving views of administration, parents, boards of control and the community. There is nearly always some element of concern that authority will perceive staff as not doing an effective job in preventing such actions.

Sex play undoubtedly occurs at any time of the year; but in residential centers in temperate climates, there does seem to be some relationship between sex play and the spring of the year. Maybe there is just greater opportunity as the children move out of more closed winter quarters to play in outdoor spaces where adult supervision is diminished. Alfred Lord Tennyson wrote in "Locksley Hall" of the relationship between spring and the turning of fancy to thoughts of love. But sexual activities among the young are motivated by several sources. Some sex play is out of curiosity, an interest in comparing anatomy; some out of the coercive use of power over another child; some as a seductive peace-making effort of one child toward another; some out of feelings of the need for intimacy and closeness to another human; some because it is a forbidden activity; and some because of its pleasurable aspects, no less. Sex play no doubt can contain several motivational elements at the same time.

With children from many diverse backgrounds and experiences and with many problems, an array of sexual attitudes and behaviors should not be unexpected. An agency has to make a decision about what its attitude will be toward various sexual behaviors. This decision will be based on several determinants—personal beliefs of the agency head as well as staff members, prevailing attitudes of the community, and the beliefs of the agency sponsors. Continuing staff discussion, not merely on a crisis basis, helps an agency clarify its views. Even so, there will be a formal or official view and an informal or unofficial view, as not everyone will agree. It is helpful for the children, though, if staff expectations are as consistent as possible. The aim should be to help the children understand their feelings whenever possible and to help them manage their feelings and behavior in a manner that is responsible to themselves and others and which is socially acceptable.

EXHIBITIONISM IN CHILDHOOD

Troubled children in group living exhibit themselves occasionally to peers and sometimes (but more rarely) to adults.

Jimmie, a boy of eight, was reported by other children to be dropping his trousers and exposing his genitalia to the girls about his age. When observed doing this one day by a child-care worker, Jimmie denied that he was exposing himself. Instead, he carefully explained that it was tick season and that the nurse had told the children to take their clothes off and examine themselves for ticks several times a day. He was seen at other times to be unfastening his trousers and attempting to show his penis, however.

Edward, another eight year old, was very hostile to his psychotherapist, a woman, as he was to most of the women on the staff. His stream of talk was filled with scatological references. In play therapy he would become quite destructive with toys, throwing them around the room. Along with this play, he would babble a steady barrage of sexual words, laughing loudly. On several occasions this behavior was climaxed by his quickly unzipping his trousers and exposing his penis.

Nellie, a seven-year-old girl, was attracted to practically any boy; and soon after admission workers began to see a pattern in her behavior. Several times a day she would single out a boy, smile and giggle, pull up her dress with one hand, her pants down with the other. This would be accompanied by skillful "bumps and grinds" of her pelvis. This kind of behavior had occurred several times when a group was off campus for some special activity. Staff became more than reluctant, sometimes refusing, to include her in external activities. Her first tangible step toward any improvement was when she said, "I'll do it in my head." Sometimes she forgot, and a fragment of a "bump and grind" would escape; but she monitored herself fairly well. The music may have played on in her head, but she soon ceased any external response.

Muffie, a small nine year old, stopped almost every boy she met, regardless of age, pulled her dress high and informed him in concise four-letter words what she would like to do with him. She objected to underpants; and early in her stay in residence, staff discovered that having her wear trousers slowed down her acts of exhibition, not by inhibition but by making it more difficult mechanically for her to accomplish.

One day at a meeting with the nurse to see a film on sex education with other group members, Muffie was loud and outspoken. When the film showed anatomical differences between boys and girls, she exclaimed, "What's the big deal about a dick? I've seen lots of them." Her overt sex talk and solicitation continued to some extent for months. Peer pressure from the other girls and the older boys ignoring her were thought to have been instrumental in helping change her behavior. She did want to be a part of the group. Her blatant talk during the movie had embarrassed the girls, and they had expressed strong disapproval which continued until her behavior improved.

Group exhibitions among pre-pubescent boys and girls can occasionally take on a ritualistic form. Such activity may start out as a teasing tag game. However, as excitement mounts the children group according to sex; and the two sides become roving bands on the playground. Apparently there are no discernible rules, and the goal of the random running about is for a girl to "flash" a boy and vice-versa. There may be "flashing" of hoped-for breasts and immature bottoms by the girls and aspiring penises and premature bottoms by the boys. This kind of game is most likely to be played around dusk which offers the participants protection from full viewing; and it also offers some protection from detection by staff members.

Perhaps remnants of this kind of childhood urge was the source of the "mooning" and "streaking" by people of all ages in the first half of the 1970's in this country. These activities were daring for the individual "mooner" or "streaker," often urged on by compatriots who enjoyed the spectacle without having to risk their own bodies.

The group games described may change complexion quickly, however, from one of provocation to one of aggression. Several members of either sex may gang up on a member of the opposite sex and cause physical, as well as emotional, trauma. In one child-care institution where the sex games had gone on apparently for some time without staff's knowledge, five girls teamed together. They isolated a boy of twelve, one girl for each limb, holding him on his back. The fifth girl sat on his chest, unfastened his trousers and "tried to pull his penis off."

Later the girls attacked another boy of twelve who had been admitted only a short time before. This boy, who was very shy, had been through several operations for undescended testicles and a severe hypospadias. He was extremely uncertain about his sexual identity. There was still another round of surgery ahead to complete the efforts at correcting the hypospadias, as the urethral opening was still on the underside of his glans penis. The girls had heard something about Reed being different "down there" from talk by some of the other boys in his cottage. The girls ambushed Reed and gave him the same treatment they had given the first boy, giggling and teasing him mercilessly until staff learned about it and intervened. The boy was humiliated and was certain that he had been further damaged.

In the individual examples of childhood exhibitionism at the beginning of this discussion, it is interesting to note that all four of the children had atrocious histories of both physical and sexual abuse by various family adults for a long time. With extensive psychiatric treatment in a residential setting, all improved in many ways including gradual disappearance of the act of exhibiting themselves. Their interpersonal relationships improved and were not nearly so threatening for them. Academic learning increased by leaps and bounds. Yet, each had a vulnerable ego from the earlier bombardment of hurtful and harmful forces.

In those "group exhibitions" which have a quality of curiosity and innocence, it is usually possible to identify the leaders. Most often they are the children, boys or girls, who have experienced an unusual amount of early sexual stimulation and sexual abuse and aggression by adults. That was the situation in the group described in which one streetwise girl of eleven, more physiologically mature than any of the boys and most of the girls, managed with consummate skill to turn more ordinary peer relationships into seductive combat.

Another example of group play which contained elements of both sex and aggression was the activity of a "Hickey Club" in a boys' residential program. Staff noted that there was a "rash" of blue and yellow marks, several millimeters in diameter, around the necks and upper chests of the nine-, ten-, and eleven-year-old boys. These marks cleared up after several days but tended to recur as isolated spots or sometimes in a chain around the neck, not unlike a necklace in configuration.

In a discussion with a ten year old who had named the club, he said, "To make a hickey, you find some skin, press your front teeth and lips against the skin, suck hard, and you will make a hickey. Do not bite; that is vampire stuff." Queried about his knowledge and expertise, he said that he used to see his father and mother make hickeys and that sometimes they got mad, bit each other and made each other bleed. "That used to scare me," he said, "because they would fight hard and hurt each other." Then he told how some of the "Hickey Club" members had fought and how one boy "got a black eye."

ADOLESCENT SEXUAL PROBLEMS

The sexual problems of adolescents in residential treatment are similar in some ways to those of younger children. But, of course, they are different in that they are more adult-like in their behaviors. The fact that they are capable of procreation adds another critical dimension. An individual's responsibility for behavior takes on new meaning. There is earlier pairing in dating now and, as mentioned, increased sexual activity. Along with these changing activities have come an increase in teenage venereal disease and an increase in teenage pregnancy.

There is no reason to think that troubled adolescents in residential care are appreciably different from other teenagers in their sexual feelings, thoughts and actions. (Many of them have little self-control, coupled with poor judgment and irresponsible attitudes.) Thus, there are potential problem areas which residential agency administration and staff must address. What are socially acceptable boundaries for adolescent boy/girl relationships in that particular agency?—that community? What is the agency position in regard to contraception, especially oral contraception (birth control pills)? Does the agency have a consulting gynecologist?—urologist? To what extent should parents or parent surrogates be involved in such decisions? What is the agency's responsible role if an adolescent has a venereal infection—gonorrhea, syphilis, venereal herpes, venereal warts, among others? These are all transmissible diseases; and severe, far-reaching complications can result from some of them.

What does an agency do when a teenage resident becomes pregnant? Where does agency responsibility begin and end for the adolescent as well as the unborn child? These are all extremely important issues with personal, interpersonal, social and ethical aspects. A residential agency for troubled adolescents cannot deny them. Examination of its reasoned positions and practices ahead of time will help when difficult decisions have to be made.

MISCELLANEOUS PROBLEMS

There are a number of medical problems which are prone to increase anxiety and activate sexual fears in children: the congenital defects of hypospadias and undescended testicles in boys; phimosis (a constrictive foreskin which interferes with cleanliness and may interfere with urination) that may require circumcision; in either sex, chronic urinary infections or other kinds of genitourinary problems that require catheterizations, instrumentations or surgical procedures in the genital area. Voiding difficulties after surgery not even related to the genitourinary tract can arouse great apprehension in children and adolescents that something has been done to their genitals. It is not unusual for a younger boy, or even a troubled adolescent, to say that he thinks he has been castrated or altered in some manner. Girls likewise, adolescents in particular, may fantasize that something has been done to change their ability to bear children. Younger children are prone to fantasize that they are being punished for transgressions of various kinds.

Sexual identity, even during adolescence, is not always a sure thing. Some adolescents fear (or even wish) for a sex-change operation; and surgical procedures of different kinds may evoke these uncertainties about sexual identity. Any examination or surgical procedure (and especially if it is related to the genitourinary system) should be explained beforehand as simply as possible and as many times as necessary. The child or adolescent must have ample opportunity to ask questions.

A STAFF'S POSSIBLE PART IN SEXUAL PROBLEMS

There may be attitudes and behaviors among staff, as well as agency practices, which make sexual problems more pronounced among children in residence. Several are listed with some brief discussion:

1. Encouraging children to act out sexual behavior because of unresolved sexual conflicts of the staff member. Such conflicts in a staff member, although on an unconscious level, can create many problems in a residential setting. Supervisors need to be alert to this possibility.

2. Telling the children stories of the staff member's sexual prowess when he or she was younger.

3. Seductive behavior toward children or adolescents by a staff member.

4. Seductive behavior between or among staff members in the presence of child residents.

5. Sexual activity in the vicinity of the children. This can occur under a variety of circumstances, such as young married couples being assigned to duty (and to sleeping quarters) in a cottage full of teenagers. In a known instance where this happened, the boys were in such a state of sexual excitement from the night sounds beyond the thin walls (and their fantasies) that they hardly slept at all. Another situation is a visit by a girlfriend or boyfriend to see a staff member on duty after the children are in bed. Visits of this kind may lead to petting or even intercourse at a time and place where it is inappropriate. Children always find out about this kind of clandestine behavior by staff and repercussions always follow.

6. The wearing of inappropriate clothing by a staff member–skin-tight clothing, transparent blouse, no brassiere, no shirt, and mini-skirts, among others may be too stimulating to children.

7. Physical handling of children, especially older ones, might be misinterpreted as sexual in nature. Children (adolescents especially) may unconsciously seek to be restrained by adults. Staff should be on the alert for the behavior may be sexually motivated, and physical encounter and restraint should be avoided if at all possible.

8. A staff member's willingness, sometimes eagerness, to be of help by taking individual children for home visits with them can cause problems of rivalry with other children, as well as profound feelings of rejection among those not taken. (There may be times when such child/staff relationships are of profound help to a child, or even a small group of children.) Some agencies have strict rules against children visiting staff in their homes and others encourage it. There are so many potential problems, however, that any agency should consider most carefully any home visiting with staff members.

When the child is an adolescent, the potential for trouble increases. In one adolescent center where staff/patient relationships were very informal, a male staff member who lived near the campus permitted the mid- to late-adolescent girls to visit his apartment in small groups when he was off duty. Sometimes one girl was seen to be visiting him alone. This was asking for trouble, which was not long in coming, in the form of accusations about sexual advances by the staff member. Whether anything sexual occurred or not, this was an unpleasant experience for all concerned. The girl was upset, and the male staff member resigned soon thereafter.

In a poorly-staffed center for early- to late-adolescent boys, a young staff member would frequently reward some particular boy with an afternoon trip or occasional overnight stay in her house in town. At other times when a boy would be upset and having frequent episodes of loss of control, she would take him to visit for a few hours of respite from his peers on campus. Her husband was there part of the time but most often was away at work. These arrangements were potentially dangerous for all concerned. Sexual fantasy was wildly stimulated in these adolescents, and there was disapproving talk in the community about an agency that allowed this amount of staff autonomy.

9. Inappropriate staffing patterns may contribute to serious problems. For example, it has happened that a young woman may be left at night with a cottage of adolescent males; and rape and accusations of rape have occurred. Likewise, a male should not be the only person left to care for a group of girls.

MANAGEMENT AND TREATMENT
OF SEXUAL PROBLEMS

In summary, the immediate management and longer-range treatment of sexual problems in a residential agency require special attitudes and skills on the part of staff. Though difficult, it is important for staff to regard sexual behavior as another form of human behavior. To the extent that staff members can do this, they will not become too emotionally involved (or threatened) and can approach solutions more rationally. "Another form of human behavior" does not suggest that an agency should not have standards and expectations of behavior. It should, for a treatment agency is one of the institutions of society that is expected to be and has to be involved in passing on the beliefs, behaviors, attitudes and practices that sustain a civilized society.

Beyond the immediate management practices aimed at protecting the children, the staff and society, a residential child agency works toward helping the children with sexual problems through its total treatment program of which psychotherapy is a vital part. Part of that total treatment view is comprised of staff attitude, example, and expectations. Appropriate sex education, individual and group, aims toward enlightenment and responsibility. There are many times and situations when medical personnel must be involved in both prevention and treatment of these problems.

The Impact
of Sexually-Stimulating Materials
and Group Care Residents:
A Question of Harm

Raymond Schimmer, MA

SUMMARY. Residential treatment center staff members frequently include provisions for management of sexually-stimulating media as part of Agency sexuality policies. This paper reviews recent attempts to calculate the impact that exposure to several categories of sexualized media has on experimental subjects. Research findings are assessed with respect to potential harm that exposure may do to youth in care, and guidelines for policy development are offered.

INTRODUCTION

Group care facility staff, in devising policies that apply to the sexual development of their residents, may become entangled when they approach the subject of sexually-stimulating materials. Immediate concerns are most troublesome, and may dominate initial discus-

This article is based on a presentation to the American Association of Children's Residential Centers Annual Meeting in October, 1990.

The author may be written at the Parsons Family and Children's Center, 60 Academy Road, Albany, NY 12208.

[Haworth co-indexing entry note]: "The Impact of Sexually-Stimulating Materials and Group Care Residents: A Question of Harm." Schimmer, Raymond. Co-published simultaneously in *Residential Treatment for Children & Youth* (The Haworth Press, Inc.) Vol. 11, No. 2, 1993, pp. 37-55; and: *The Management of Sexuality in Residential Treatment* (ed: Gordon Northrup) The Haworth Press, Inc., 1993, pp. 37-55. Multiple copies of this article/chapter may be purchased from The Haworth Document Delivery Center [1-800-3-HAWORTH; 9:00 a.m. - 5:00 p.m. (EST)].

sion: should residents be allowed to display pin-ups, to subscribe to sexually-oriented magazines, to attend "R-rated" movies, and if not, why not? How intrusive should staff be, particularly when dealing with older residents?

These questions lead surely to another that is broader and more fundamental. What manner of harm, if any, befalls young people in care as a consequence of exposure to such materials? A clear answer simultaneously establishes the responsibility to act and the justification for doing so; however, clear answers on this topic have been elusive.

This paper explores contemporary social science research and attempts to relate some of the relevant data to group care policy and practice. It looks at findings concerning the impact of sexually-stimulating materials as presented in two recent, major surveys: the *Attorney General's Commission on Pornography: Final Report* (1986),[1] and *The Question of Pornography: Research Findings and Implications* (1987)[2] by Edward Donnerstein, Daniel Linz and Steven Penrod.

The Attorney General's Commission accepted a broad charge ("...we were asked to determine the nature, extent, and impact on society of pornography in the United States."),[3] and noted that it was underfinanced,[4] and understaffed; nevertheless, it conducted extensive public hearings, reviewed nearly 300 research reports, and also examined hundreds of other related documents.

Donnerstein et al. looked extensively into similar areas and included approximately 800 sources in their bibliography. Their intent was simple: " . . . to give the reader the most up-to-date summary of the scientific research on the effects of sexually explicit images on anti-social attitudes and behaviors."[5]

Throughout this paper, the term "sexually stimulating material" is used to refer to any media depiction that has the potential to arouse reviewers sexually. The definition is purposely broad, because the daily exposure of young people to potentially arousing images and portrayals is now, for better or worse, a characteristic of contemporary culture. Edward Donnerstein (1989) summarized this condition in a recent interview:

> We say that certain messages have negative effects. The problem is that these messages are all over the place, not just in

pornography. For example, a recent *Time* magazine advertisement for an ABC show about a woman who fell in love with the man who raped her and killed her husband. What we're trying to say is that violent forms of pornography have that message, but, unfortunately, so does all the media.[6]

BACKGROUND: THE QUESTION OF HARM

Governments have long been concerned with the concept of harm and sexually-stimulating material. They have historically presumed that a depiction of lewd erotic activity enervated the citizenry, and contributed to a general laxity that would ultimately erode the foundation of civilized behavior. Such depictions were believed to de-personalize sexuality, and to coarsen in general the interactions between male and female. They were seen as facilitating the development of a dangerously self-centered, regressive world-view on the part of individual citizens. Lord Justice Powell, presiding over an obscenity trial in 1708, spoke for many who would follow him when he offered his opinion about the effects of sexualized literature " . . . It indeed tends to the corruption of good manners."[7] Many public-minded Victorians accepted this proposition completely and acted vigorously upon it. By 1890, the United States had enacted a sizable canon of Federal obscenity law, amended vestiges of which are still operative today. This law was intended to protect individuals and the national character from the harm presumed to be directly caused by sexually-stimulating material.

During the Twentieth Century, Americans began considering a new type of harm—that done to free speech and the First Amendment by obscenity legislation. Even if obscenity were harmful to individuals and ultimately to the society, would prosecuting it cause even greater harm to a way of life predicated on the free flow of ideas and information? Over a period of seventy years, through a series of celebrated cases, the Supreme Court established four principles that currently structure legal activity in this area:

a. The First Amendment " . . . cannot have been, and obviously was not, intended to give immunity for every possible use of language" (Frohwerk vs. U.S., 1919).[8]

b. Obscenity, lewd offensive speech and "fighting words" are not protected by the First Amendment (Chaplinsky vs. U.S., 1932).[9]

c. There is a definition of obscenity (Miller vs. California, 1973).[10]

d. Obscenity as defined may be prosecuted by states and localities (Paris Adult Theater I vs. Slaton, 1973).[11]

In short, the Court thinks that there is such a thing as obscenity, that it is worthless, and that it does not merit the protection of the First Amendment.

But the Supreme Court has not defined obscenity as harmful, only utterly without merit. After all the many decisions, the toxicity of obscenity was still only a subject of speculation, and not a proven fact.

In 1970, President Richard Nixon appointed a Commission on Obscenity and Pornography. The Commission was instructed to investigate the effect of sexually-explicit material on behavior. The Commission's establishment marked the first time the scientific methodology would be trained systematically on the question of harm. It would be the forerunner of several more foreign and domestic inquiries.

The Commission was given a budget of $2,000,000, with which it funded 80 independent studies. These were completed in less than two years, and were the basis of a very controversial summary. Among the Commission's conclusions were these:

> [There is] no substantial basis for the belief that erotic materials constitute a primary or significant cause of the development of character deficit . . . it is not possible to conclude that erotic material is a significant cause of crime.[12]

> [There is] no support for the thesis that experience with sexual materials is a significant factor in the cause of juvenile delinquency.[13]

> . . . the data do not appear to support the thesis of a causal connection between increased availability of erotica and the commission of sex offenses . . . [14]

The Commission recommended that in light of its findings, there was no need for an increase in legislation or prosecution. Its investigation had not found evidence of harm. The Commission acquitted the defendant.

President Nixon was not pleased with his Commission: "I have evaluated that report and categorically reject its morally bankrupt conclusions and major recommendations."[15] Many others as well accused the Commission of having a liberal bias that blinded it to the true nature of erotica. Critics noted that the Commission's studies were conducted in less than two years–scarcely enough time to provide a comprehensive or in-depth analysis. They wondered why, if the Surgeon General could link exposure to violent images and behavior in the impact of television violence,[16] the Commission was completely unable to find links between exposure to sexual images and behavior.

Part of the answer to the latter criticism is that the Commission was not looking at the admixture of sex and violence. It concentrated its work on sexually-explicit, non-violent materials, referring to them as "erotica" and "sexual materials." In its short lifetime, the Committee did not attempt to categorize types of images, and eventually made rather broad pronouncements that may have been to some degree misleading in light of later research.

Criticism not withstanding, the *Report* was in fact a significant initial effort to organize an extremely confused field and bring to bear scientific methodology on it. The report stood as the major work on sexually-explicit imagery and consequent behavior through most of the decade.

By the late 1970's, anti-pornography forces had regrouped. Conservative politicians, now ascendent, joined in an unlikely coalition with radical feminists to propose sweeping restrictive legislation. The conservatives resurrected their traditional arguments. The anti-pornography feminists, on the other hand, presented a new and profoundly expanded concept of harm. They defined pornography broadly, and held that its existence was fundamental to the denial of civil rights and equal opportunity to all women in the country. Catharine MacKinnon, who was a leader in the development of an anti-pornography ordinance in Minneapolis, summarized this argument: ". . . pornography causes attitudes and behaviors of violence and discrimination which define the treatment of half the population."[17] Pornography–in this definition including even the simple depiction of female body parts–caused the attitudes and behavior that bring about the violent subjugation of women. Pornography's existence symbolized unwarranted sexual domination, but more importantly, was responsible for real events and real injuries. Pornography was a significant cause of suppression of a entire class of people as defined by sex, and as such it constituted harm on a scale previously unconsidered.

Although this new coalition achieved mixed success legislatively, it did return the subject of pornography to the national stage. Research efforts were redoubled, and in 1985, President Reagan appointed the government's second blue-ribbon study group, later known as the Meese Commission.

REVIEW OF SOCIAL SCIENCE RESEARCH

Before looking at the literature, it is important to understand some of its limitations. One understates in saying that the field is controversial. The Canadian government's "Fraser Committee" on pornography and prostitution addresses this quality clearly, if harshly:

> ... the research is so inadequate and chaotic that no consistent body of information has been established. However, overall, the results of the research are contradictory and inconclusive.[18]

This, and similar opinion, derives at least in part to the current state of research methodology. With a few notable exceptions, most studies do not report on behavior in the natural environment. They instead describe what happens in laboratories under very specific conditions, and it is difficult to make determinations about real life behavior on the basis of laboratory experimentation. Donnerstein et al.'s own description of a typical experiment provides telling detail. Experiment subjects are almost always undergraduate college students. They are intentionally misled about the true nature of the experiment. The subjects are asked to perform a task, and are irritated by other students (confederates of the experimenter) who grade them poorly and who may administer mild electric shocks to the subjects as "punishment" for poor performance. Having "primed" the subjects to egress, the experimenter declares a break, during which a sub-set of the subjects is exposed to some type of sexually-stimulating material. After the break, the subjects get to evaluate and "punish" the confederates. The intensity of the "punishment" administered by the experiment subjects is considered an index of their aggression, and is compared with that of the control group which has not been shown any sexually-stimulating materials.

The problems here are evident: the collegiate experimental group is not representative of the general population; the experiment depends on the subjects being unaware of the true nature of the experiment; and the punishment administered by the subjects is only presumed to be an accurate index of their emotional state and behavioral capability.

Donnerstein et al. offer a convincing defense of the methodology, but acknowledge that experimental findings are only directly relevant to the lab situations. One extrapolates from them at one's peril. Donnerstein et al. warn:

> ... as researchers we would be hard-pressed to derive a set of rules for regulating pornographic materials on the basis of empirical inquiries so far. At best, we are able to specify what types of materials result in given effects (with some of these effects generally regarded as harmful and others more questionably so) and under what conditions the effects are more likely to occur.[19]

In addition to these particular problems, standard research difficulties are also at play. Methodology may be flawed; similar experiments often produce contradictory findings; and unexpected or unidentified variables may influence outcomes. These reservations should be kept in mind when attempting to evaluate the literature.

Arousal Following Exposure to Sexually-Stimulating Material

The President's Commission (1970) confirmed common knowledge: exposure to sexually-stimulating materials tends to arouse most adults. The arousal can be measured physiologically. Males tend to be more aroused by visual images, females by literature. Howard, Reifler and Liptzen,[20] working for the President's Commission, found that repeated exposure seemed to induce boredom: after eight weeks of exposure to sexually explicit movies, subjects were less aroused physiologically by the materials and less interested in them. They also altered their attitudes about pornography, regarding it as less harmful than they had previously. The Commission's researchers found a minor sexual behavioral correlate to exposure: there seemed to be a brief (24 hours) period of increased sexual activity for subjects who were already sexual partners, but there appeared to be no behavioral changes in those participants who were not already involved in a sexual relationship. Zillmann and Bryant (1984)[21] expanded on this base, showing that subjects massively exposed to erotica over six weeks responded with less aggression, lower heart-rates, less repulsion and more enjoyment than did groups less frequently exposed.

Although simple arousal does not appear to have significant behavioral consequences, these may develop under certain circumstances. When a subject is exposed to erotica while in a pronounced state of anger or irritation, increased aggression toward both same and opposite sexes may occur, as described below. Donnerstein et al., citing research by Zillman et al.,[22] emphasize that it is the physical and emotional arousal, not the particular stimulant (e.g., exposure to sexually explicit material) that actualizes the aggression. Noise, physical exercise, and even humor have also been found to generate aggression-facilitating arousal.

Exposure to Depictions of Violent Sexual Behavior

If there is any point on which there is general agreement among researchers, it is that exposure to material mixing sex and violence can produce aggressive behavior in viewers.

> The most well-documented finding in the social science literature is that all sexually violent material in our society, whether sexually explicit or not, tends to promote aggression against women. (Donnerstein et al., 1981)[23]

> When clinical and experimental research has focused primarily on sexually violent material, the conclusions have been

virtually unanimous . . . exposure to sexually violent materials has indicated an increase in the likelihood of aggression. (Attorney General's Commission: Final Report, 1986)[24]

One study in particular demonstrates the connection between sexually-violent material and consequent aggression. Malamuth (1978)[25] had one group of male undergraduates read a neutral story, another read a sexual but non-violent story, and a third read a story about rape. All subjects were angered by female research confederates, and were then placed in a situation in which they could "aggress" upon the women. Half of all the subjects were given permission to aggress ("disinhibited") and half were discouraged from aggressing. The "disinhibited" males who had read the rape story were significantly more aggressive than any of the other five groups. Donnerstein and Berkowitz (1981)[26] then produced similar results using similar methodology.

Many violently sexual depictions express or imply a positive outcome for the victim; i.e., the victim ultimately derives pleasure from the assault. This common presentation may in fact facilitate disinhibition. The victim's positive response extends permission to the viewer to be aggressive by saying that forcible sex is what the victim actually wants, her superficial protestations notwithstanding. The viewer, reinforced by the victim, and already identifying with the media perpetrator, is thus strongly induced to shed inhibitions.

"Positive" victim outcomes in such material may also be responsible for those attitudinal changes associated with exposure to sexually-violent material. The Attorney General's *Final Report* describes attitudes that appear to become measurably stronger in viewers after exposure:

a. viewers perceive rape victims as more responsible for their victimization;
b. viewers perceive victims as having suffered less, and having been less degraded;
c. rapists are perceived as being less responsible and less deserving of punishment; and
d. viewers accept components of the "rape myth" more readily. They believe more strongly that women enjoy coercion, pain

and degradation, and that women's resistance is superficial and not indicative of their true feelings.

The Commission shared Donnerstein et al.'s opinion that the degree of sexual explicitness is not the essential component in producing laboratory aggression and attitudinal change. The culprit appears to be the juxtaposition of sex–however explicit–and violence. R-rated "slasher" films are regarded as particularly insidious:

> ... the so-called 'slasher' films ... are likely to produce the consequences discussed here to a greater extent than most of the materials available in 'adult only' pornographic outlets. (Attorney General's Commission: Final Report, 1986)[27]

Donnerstein et al. summarize the understanding of exposure to sexually violent material as follows:

> On the basis of what we knew so far, we have to assert that the kind of film that is most dangerous would be that which depicts sexual violence against women in either a sexually explicit or non-sexually explicit manner, where the victims are shown enjoying or somehow benefiting from the treatment. Furthermore, we might expect that young male adolescents who are in the process of exploring their own sexuality or beginning to date might be most affected by the material. This group might be more inclined than others to turn to the media for ideas about the appropriateness of certain sexual behaviors. (Donnerstein et al., 1987)[28]

There is some indication that the effects of exposure to this material may be temporary with respect to aggression. Malamuth and Cenuti (1986)[29] found that when they interposed a one-week delay after exposure and then reinstituted the anger situation, their subjects' level of aggression had lapsed back into the normal range, and was indistinguishable from the no-exposure control group. Donnerstein et al. conclude:

> For the moment. . . we do not know if repeated exposure to violent pornography has a cumulative effect in producing

aggression, or if such effects are only temporary. This is one area where additional research is definitely needed. We can say with certainty that there is an immediate effect, however short-lived. (Donnerstein et al., 1987)[30]

Donnerstein et al. then move to a consideration of the potential effects on viewer sensibilities that repeated exposure to sexualized violence may be having. Using desensitization theory as a point of reference, they speculate that repeated exposure reduces the amount of viewer anxiety generated by sexually violent images, which in turn may reduce viewer responsiveness and ability to empathize with victims of sexual violence:

If this proves to be true, we risk the possibility that many members of our society, particularly young viewers, will evolve into less sensitive and responsive individuals as a result, at least partly, of repeated exposure to violent media, particularly sexually violent media. (Donnerstein et al., 1987)[31]

Exposure to Sexually Non-Violent, Degrading and Dehumanizing Material

The Attorney General's Commission opened commentary on this section by explaining that it had sympathy with the widely-held view that there could be no commercialized, sexually-stimulating material that was *not* degrading and humiliating, particularly since the overwhelming majority of it is made by men using women for men's pleasure. The Commission was then strong and clear on the subject: exposure to materials depicting degradation, domination, subordination or humiliation are harmful on a large scale. The Commision felt that the research established that individual viewers are affected negatively, and that the moral, ethical, and cultural harm comes to the larger society as well. The Commission made a jump that others felt unsubstantiated—it extrapolated from lab research to make assertions about actual behavior:

. . . we conclude that substantial exposure to materials of this type bears some causal relationship to the level of sexual violence, sexual coercion, or unwanted sexual aggression in the population so exposed. (Attorney General's Commission: Final Report, 1986)[32]

The Commission also attributed the same attitudinal changes that it associated with sexually violent material to non-violent degrading material, and described as well a measurable, increased level of sexual callousness in males exposed to degrading depictions.

Donnerstein et al. do not concur with the Commission, asserting that the evidence is "very inconsistent," and that even if it were not, the Commission errs in making declarations about real life activity that are based on laboratory events.

Non-Violent, Non-Degrading Material

This category includes images of consensual activity apparently enjoyed by all participants with disadvantage to none. The Commission and Donnerstein et al. are in substantial agreement here: there appears to be no convincing evidence indicating subsequent viewer aggressiveness or negative attitudinal change. The Commission did engage in speculation that it acknowledged to be non-scientific, but which is of some importance nonetheless.

> Intuitively and not experimentally, we can hypothesize that materials portraying such an activity will either help to legitimize or will bear some causal relationship to that activity itself. (Attorney General's Commission: Final Report, 1986)[33]

The Commission is referring here to uncommitted sexuality and promiscuity, and perhaps as well to the medical dangers of the unprotected sexual activity depicted or implied in sexual fantasy material. The Commission clearly feels that portrayals of a sexually utopian nature are problematic because of their potential for generalization in a non-utopian world. Viewers may identify with actors, reduce inhibitions, and assume that media depictions are accurate and realistic. This effect may in turn produce increased amounts of problematic sexual behavior.

Nudity

Once again, the Commission and Donnerstein et al. are in general agreement. Both sources regard depiction of simple nudity as essentially harmless. As noted earlier, some research exists that indicates the type of mild erotic effect engendered by such depictions may actually reduce aggression. The Commission, however, qualified its position:

> We are concerned about the impact of such material on children, on attitudes toward women, on the relationship between the sexes, and on attitudes towards sex in general, but the extent of the harms was the subject of some difference of opinion. (Attorney General's Commission: Final Report, 1986)[34]

The Commission's reservations here probably apply to that common example of sexually-stimulatory material, the pin-up. The Commission obviously feels that there is a potential for difficulty even in this, the most benign of the four categories.

RESEARCH CONCLUSION

The following generalizations seem to enjoy substantial research support:

a. Exposure to sexually-explicit materials while subjects are predisposed to aggression tends to elicit aggressive behavior immediately after exposure in laboratory situations.
b. Exposure to sexually violent material in circumstances described above results in significantly greater rates of laboratory aggression than does exposure to other types of sexual material.
c. Sexually violent and sexually degrading materials tend to elicit aggression and alter attitudes toward women. Viewers become more calloused about victim suffering, and embrace to a greater degree components of the "rape myth."

d. Many "R" rated materials, and materials otherwise considered non-obscene, contain juxtapositions of sex and violence that facilitate aggression and attitude changes as described above.

e. Simple exposure to non-violent, non-degrading sexual depictions, irrespective of their explicitness, does not appear to cause increased viewer aggression or attitudinal changes in laboratory situations.

f. Mild erotica, including simple nudity, does not appear to cause behavioral or attitudinal changes in viewers.

g. Sexual offenders and rapists may respond differentially to sexually-stimulating materials. Offenders have been observed to become more physiologically aroused by sexual depictions than non-offenders. Convicted rapists appear less aroused by sexually-explicit materials, but significantly more aroused by violent depictions, with or without sexual content.

Although the Attorney General's Commission and Donnerstein et al. agree in large part on the above statements, they disagree directly in their conclusions. The Commission appeared to be strongly influenced by the feminist thinkers, going so far as to quote Robin Morgan's famous statement: "Pornography is the theory; rape is the practice," in its report.[35] The Commission's chief recommendation was to increase legislation and intensify prosecution. It had found that harm was involved, and that it was sufficiently serious to warrant vigorous government involvement.

Donnerstein et al. do not believe that the case for harm has yet been made decisively. They feel that the leap from laboratory to legislation is precipitous. They are, to be sure, greatly impressed by the problematic potential of sexually violent material, but point out that violence, not sex, seems to be the active agent in the production of negative effects. They also note that much sexually violent material is not legally obscene. Legislation may be irrelevant and may in fact distract attention from the problem of violence.

COMMENTARY ON RESEARCH

For the purposes of group care management, the body of research on sexually stimulating media is presently underdeveloped. For example, little work has been done to describe different effects among discrete viewer categories, aside from preliminary work with sex offenders and rapists. Categories for future study could profitably include victims of sex abuse, juvenile sex offense perpetrators, developmentally disabled and retarded adolescents and adults, etc. However, the ethical problem concerning child research may be insurmountable—one simply cannot show sexually stimulating material to children to see what will happen. At this point, we can only speculate about the effects of such exposure on specific groups of clients often found in residential care. Most importantly, the scientific literature is sparse with respect to exposure to stimulating images and depictions that surround adolescents in daily life. Donnerstein et al. note:

> It should be obvious to everyone with a television set that mass-media contain an abundance of violent non-sexually explicit (and thus non-obscene) images and messages. These ideas about rape and sexual violence may be so pervasive in our culture that it is myopic to call them the exclusive domain of violent pornography, much less the domain of the broader category of legally obscene materials. (Donnerstein et al., 1987)[36]

Exposure to what has traditionally been known as pornography may not be the most serious threat to object relations, self-esteem, and instinctual-impulse control. That may instead be the profusion of daily images that is all the more insidious because of its banality. Knowledge about the impact of mundane exposure will illuminate both management practice and clinical treatment.

Existing research tends to focus on aggression, criminal behavior, and associated attitudes. Additional work is needed on other behaviors, including promiscuity and uncommitted sexuality in general. These seem particularly relevant in light of the AIDS threat and the increase in prevalence of sexually transmitted diseases.

Finally, none of the research cited by the Attorney General or Donnerstein et al., dealt with aural material. The point may be a minor one, but substantial amounts of explicit sexual description, sado-masochism, and sexual violence are presented to adolescents through audio tapes. The effects of these materials on young people seem to be largely undocumented.

Despite its shortcomings, the body of existing research has made possible several important developments. It has moved dialogue on the question of harm beyond political and moral contexts and to more objective ground. Although passionate subjectivity will probably always have its place in the discussion, the scientific method is a desirable complement. The existing research has also helped to move the focus of concern from "pornography" and sexual-explicitness to the mixture of sexual and violent imagery. It makes clear that our traditional pre-occupation with sexual depiction may well be leading us away from a more potently harmful genre of media representation. Lastly, the research is giving us some inkling of what exactly happens when people are exposed to sexually-stimulating material. Although far from complete, the scientific inquiry has already provided us with a level of detail that was previously unavailable.

POLICY DEVELOPMENT

The following suggestions may be useful in the development of policies that regulate the use of sexually-stimulating media by residents within a group care context.

1. Process policies thoroughly with staff. The subject is controversial for many reasons, and conflicting opinions abound.

2. Seriously consider research findings relative to exposure to sexual violence and its apparent effects on behavior and attitude. Clearly, the research must be regarded carefully, but the apparently strong findings in this particular area warrant special attention. Violence, alone and in combination with sexual depictions, is probably of more concern than is simple explicitness. Residences would most likely do well to prohibit such material because of the possible danger that it holds for young people. Prohibitions should focus especially on sex-violence combinations, even if they are not pornographic or obscene.

3. Consider research on sexually-degrading material as it relates

to the individual in possession of it, and also as it relates to other individuals who may see such material or know of its existence on a unit. Residential staff must be aware that such material may contribute to an atmosphere of sexual threat and intimidation.

4. Articulate reasons for all points of policy, and be ready to discuss them openly with residents. The two principal points supporting restrictions are: there is reason to believe that exposure to sexually-violent and degrading materials may affect the quality of inter-personal relationships; and the presence of such materials may insult or intimidate others, including staff members. The underlying theme is not that such materials are abstractly evil in a vague way, but that they are specifically bad for specific human beings.

5. Anticipate potential secondary effects of restrictions. These may include:
   a. a tendency of residents to "go underground" and thereby remove themselves from clinical interventions;
   b. feelings by residents that their unique, personal strengths and needs are being discounted—that their ability to manage such material without harm and without staff help is not being recognized.

6. Train staff members to use questions or complaints about the policy as educational opportunities. Staff members should be able to explain that sexually violent material may impair a youth's ability to relate successfully to others, and that various forms or explicit material may offend others.

7. Apprise families and other parties with custody of clients concerning the Agency's policy. The policy is in fact a statement of values that may not be shared by all of the many client cultures. These people need to know what guidelines residential staff are using in caring for their children.

8. Be aware that a young person's involvement with stimulating materials may have diagnostic implications. Staff members should assess the amount and quality of interest in the material, as well as the content of the material. Individualized plans should be considered for youth with histories of sexually aggressive behavior, or who have been victimized sexually.

BIBLIOGRAPHY

Attorney General's Commission on Pornography: Final Report. Washington, D.C.: U.S. Department of Justice, July 1986.

Commission on Obscenity and Pornography. *The report of the commission on obscenity and pornography.* Washington, D.C.: U.S. Government Printing Office, 1970.

Donnerstein, E.; Linz, D. and Penrod, S. *The question of pornography: Research findings and implications.* New York: The Free Press, 1987.

Downs, D.A. *The new politics of pornography.* Chicago, IL: The University of Chicago Press, 1989.

REFERENCES

1. *Attorney General's Commission on Pornography: Final Report.* Washington, D.C.: U.S. Department of Justice, July 1986.

2. Donnerstein, E.; Linz, D. and Penrod, S. *The question of pornography: Research findings and implications.* New York: The Free Press, 1987.

3. *Attorney General's Commission on Pornography: Final Report,* p. 215.

4. The Attorney General's Commission had a budget of $500,000 for one year; the President's Commission in 1970 operated with $2,000,000 for two years.

5. Donnerstein et al., p. 215.

6. Downs, D.A. *The new politics of pornography.* Chicago, IL: The University of Chicago Press, 1989, pp. 189-190.

7. Queen vs. Read. Fortestcue Reports 98, 92 Eng. Rep. 777 (1708).

8. Frohwerk vs. United States 249, U.S. 204 (1919).

9. Chaplinsky vs. United States (1932).

10. Miller vs. California, 413, U.S. 15 (1973).

11. Paris Adult Theatre I vs. Slaton 413, U.S. 49 (1973).

12. Commission on Obscenity and Pornography. *The report of the commission on obscenity and pornography.* Washington D.C.: U.S. Government Printing Office, 1970, p. 243.

13. Commission on Obscenity and Pornography, 1970, p. 255.

14. Commission on Obscenity and Pornography, 1970, p. 229.

15. Rist, R.C. *The pornography controversy: Changing moral standards in American life.* New Brunswick, NJ: Transaction Books, 1975. In Donnerstein et al., 1987, p. 35.

16. Surgeon General's Scientific Advisory Committee on Television and Social Behavior. *Television and growing up: The impact of televised violence.* Washington, D.C.: U.S. Government Printing Office, 1972.

17. MacKinnon, C. Pornography, civil right and speech: Commentary. *Harvard Civil Rights–Civil Liberties Law Review,* 1985 (20) pp. 1-70. In Donnerstein et al., p. 141.

18. *Report of the special committee on pornography and prostitution.* N.I. Ottawa: Ministry of Supply and Services, 1985. In Donnerstein et al.

19. Donnerstein et al., pp. 144.

20. Howard, J.L.; Reifler, C.B. and Liptzen, M.B. Effects of exposure to pornography. In *Technical report of the commission on obscenity and pornography* (Vol. 8). Washington, D.C.: U.S. Government Printing Office, 1970. In Donnerstein et al., p. 29.

21. Zillman, D. and Bryant, J. Effects of massive exposure to pornography. In Malamuth, N. and Donnerstein, E. (Eds.) *Pornography and sexual aggression.* In Donnerstein et al., pp. 49-50.

22. Zillman, D.; Bryant, J.; Comisky, P.W. and Medoff, N.J. Excitation and hedonic valence in the effect of erotica on motivated intermale aggression. *European Journal of Social Psychology,* 1981 (11), pp. 233-252, in Donnerstein et al., p. 47.

23. Donnerstein et al., 1987, p. 179.

24. Attorney General's Commission: Final Report, 1986, p. 324.

25. Malamuth, N. *Erotica, aggression and perceived appropriateness.* Paper presented at the annual meeting of the American Psychological Association, Toronto, September 1978. In Donnerstein et al., 1987.

26. Donnerstein, E. and Berkowitz, L. Victim reactions in aggressive erotic films as a factor in violence against women. *Journal of Personality and Social Psychology,* 1981 (41) pp. 710-724. In Donnerstein et al., 1987, p. 94.

27. Attorney General's Commission: Final Report, 1986, p. 329.

28. Donnerstein et al., p. 160.

29. Malamuth, N. and Cenuti, J. Repeated exposure to violent and non-violent pornography: Likelihood of raping ratings and laboratory aggressive against women. *Aggressive Behavior,* 1986 (12), pp. 129-137. In Donnerstein et al., 1986, p. 99.

30. Donnerstein et al., p. 100.

31. Donnerstein et al., p. 136.

32. Attorney General's Commission: Final Report, 1986, p. 334.

33. Attorney General's Commission: Final Report, 1986, p. 338.

34. Ibid, p. 348.

35. Attorney General's Commission: Final Report, 1986, p. 78.

36. Donnerstein et al., 1987, pp. 178-179.

Discovery and Treatment
of Adolescent Sexual Offenders
in a Residential Treatment Center

Richard Burnett, MSSW, ACSW
Cheryl Rathbun, MSW

SUMMARY. This paper describes how a facility came to understand the pervasiveness of physical and sexual abuse among its male adolescent conduct disorder population. A major decision was whether sexual offenders should or could be treated in a heterogeneous (non-offender) population. Security and liability became administrative, treatment, transference, and countertransference issues. In addition, there was the need for a trial and error development of a treatment protocol for this modality. There were both successes and failures. Follow-up research, two years post-treatment, is reported.

TREATING ADOLESCENT SEXUAL OFFENDERS
IN A RESIDENTIAL TREATMENT CENTER

Saint Francis at Ellsworth, a related corporation to The Saint Francis Academy, Incorporated, serves 26 boys, twelve to seventeen years of age, diagnosed Conduct Disorder.

Mr. Burnett may be written at The St. Francis Academy, PO Box 1340, Salina, KS 67402-1340.

[Haworth co-indexing entry note]: "Discovery and Treatment of Adolescent Sexual Offenders in a Residential Treatment Center." Burnett, Richard and Cheryl Rathbun. Co-published simultaneously in *Residential Treatment for Children & Youth* (The Haworth Press, Inc.) Vol. 11, No. 2, 1993, pp. 57-64; and: *The Management of Sexuality in Residential Treatment* (ed: Gordon Northrup) The Haworth Press, Inc., 1993, pp. 57-64. Multiple copies of this article/chapter may be purchased from The Haworth Document Delivery Center [1-800-3-HAWORTH; 9:00 a.m. - 5:00 p.m. (EST)].

57

We know our treatment is effective (Burdsal, Force, & Klingspom, 1989; Klingspom, Force, & Burdsal, 1990). Nevertheless, about 20-30% of outcomes were not successful. In response to a follow-up contact, a former patient incarcerated for child abuse wrote: "If you'll deal with your young men on their home life. . . really see if they were abused . . . . Whether it's physical or mental or sexual it's all abuse . . . . Mine was physical. Yet I didn't want to admit it or deal with it, nor did I want to get anyone in trouble . . . I only hope to help you reach another young man before he ends up here such as I have."

Our approach had been to play down adolescent sexuality because it was probably too stimulating. We focused on current behavior and viewed historical trauma as excuses, e.g., "my father was a drunk so I stole cars." We viewed some trauma reports as fantasy based upon transferential issues. Staff felt the need for more expertise.

We employed a clinical psychologist with a background in adolescent sexuality. She enlisted the help of the Unit's psychiatric nurse and a Vietnam veteran counselor who had been treated for some Post-Traumatic Stress Disorder (PTSD) issues and was now leading a self-help group. They attended various workshops on sexuality as related to PTSD and offending. Meanwhile, we began to ask questions regarding sexuality and history at staffings. We maneuvered individual therapy sessions to be sexually focused. We bantered about the usual and some unusual four-letter words. We transferred the sex education component to direct service staff and presented the component at staffings. We made discussion of physical abuse and sexuality part of our daily culture.

Patient issues began surfacing, and we identified enough sexual offenders to commence our first group.

SEXUAL OFFENDER TREATMENT

Presenting offenses include indecent exposure, obscene telephone calls/peeping, child molestation, incest, and rape. Most presented with one to three separate victims. Approximately 70% admitted having more victims ranging from one to eight. Approximately 90% admitted to more actual offenses, ranging from a one-time offense with one victim to approximately three times a week over a one- to two-year period with one or more victims. Approximately 75% of offenders have been victims of sex abuse. Of the remaining 25%, many were exposed to an upbringing with confusing sexual messages, i.e., pornography, parents engaging in promiscuous sex in front of the child, father sexually abusive to mother in front of the child, etc.

We limited the program to ten patients for two reasons: staff felt this was the maximum they could treat, and being a minority of the total, therefore less of a threat to the milieu.

Treatment Approach

Group therapy provides a safe environment to explore sexual offense and share victimization. Self-esteem can be restored through group support and mirroring. Groups facilitate self-awareness, mutual concern, and empathy. Group therapy affords an opportunity to abreact family experiences. Peer group pressure undoes denial and minimization, as well as teaching and practicing techniques to allow the sex offender to be at lower risk to re-offend. Male and female co-therapists model parent and sex roles, working democratically, and sharing disagreement with continued respect.

Individual counseling is adjunctive to helping prepare for group, discussing non-group issues, and processing beyond the individual involvement in group. Other related individual issues include emotional literacy, journal writing, letters of clarification to the victim, and working through the offender's victimization.

Journal writing includes daily entries commenting on a variety of feelings and ideas, focusing on sexual thoughts, anger situations and plans for revenge, sexual fantasy, detailing sexual offenses, feelings about family, and empathy for the victims of sex abuse. It is a difficult task for adolescent conduct disorders to complete because it requires great discipline, and because many do not understand feelings other than that of anger.

Sex education focuses on sexual expectations, male/female anatomy, contraception, pregnancy, masturbation, and same sex and opposite sex relationships. We recommend male and female co-teaching.

Family therapy. The patient should not be present with the family victim until he owns the sexual offense. The family must accomplish many tasks: matter-of-factly recall the abuse, work with it emotionally and intellectually; focus on ways the patient and family can restore themselves; learn communication in different ways; accept responsibility for being secretive; love and touch in non-sexual and sexually appropriate ways; develop an equitable system of discipline; respect privacy and boundaries; have activities outside the home as a family and as an individual; learn to disagree and resolve disagreements; talk about sex (parents need education how to be teachers); go beyond sex role stereotypes, i.e., boys can cook and clean, and girls can be assertive; trust each other, talk, and have family meetings; and treat victim and offender as normally as developmental stage permits, and as normal as possible within family roles.

Reunification of the family may not be possible if all members are not able to go past the denial stage. The victim must be able to say "no," and be supported by family members.

Phases in Treatment

Assessment. The two most important criteria: inappropriate age difference, and coercion. We use a protocol from Groth and Loredo (1981) for evaluation of sexual offense: age difference between the persons involved; social relationship between the persons involved; type of sexual activity exhibited; how does the act take place; persistency of activity; evidence of progression in regard to the nature/frequency of the activity; nature of fantasies preceding or accompanying abusive behavior; and distinguishing characteristics of target of the assaults.

Orientation to the institution, its rules, and the program's expectations and ability to control and care for the patient. This facilitates peer relationships, incorporates the group into the patient's processing of rules, and facilitates staff relationships.

Undoing the denial. Defense mechanisms usually are denial, minimizing the offense, avoiding discussing the offense, distorting the facts of the offense, and/or projecting the blame and responsibility for the offense. The offender must feel safe to realign his defenses, and must be taught responsibility and coping. Confrontation must be constant, but gentle. During this process, the patient is encouraged to detail his offenses, constantly talk about them, and have peers confront him.

Each sex offender group begins with a history of the offense. Members role-play offenses, mirror feelings, and provide support for each other. As the patient relates offenses, group members identify rituals and warning signals. There is a strong focus on thinking errors (thoughts or statements which minimize, rationalize, justify, excuse, or deny the true extent of the problem, feeling, or behavior) which contribute to sexual offending.

The offender as a victim. As the patient expresses verbal and behavioral ownership of his behavior, he is encouraged to share the abuse he suffered and take risks with the pain, hurt, and trauma of being a victim himself. Working through his own victimizations is a beginning step toward empathy for victims. The patient has issues of loss, abandonment by parents, rejection by others, and loss of family due to the offense.

Skill deficit retraining. Deficits usually include social skills (assertiveness, fair fighting, conflict resolution/negotiation), boundaries, values clarification, communication skills, developing relationships, sex education, and dealing with anger feelings.

Clarification with the victim is not always possible. The patient continues to work with this process in treatment and prepare for it just as if he were to do it in person. It is not a time to apologize to the victim, but rather clarify the responsibility of the sexual offense. Clarification is accomplished through role-playing with other offenders, and journal writing. Preparation is made for greeting the victim, describing the victim as a unique and precious human being, and saying, "This is how I imagine I hurt you," thereby giving power to the victim. The offender must practice what it would be like for the victim on the day of the clarification, to be matter of fact in regard to the offense with the sensitivity of the victim in mind. The patient is prepared to answer questions from the victim and take ownership of arousal and selfishness issues. Forgiveness of the offender only gives power back to the offender. This clarification session must also occur with the offender's parents and siblings. If the victim is involved, he or she has a right to have the sessions accomplished as he or she wants. Never make the victim walk into the room with the offender there. The victim may refuse the session, as everything is in their control. If the victim is a family member and the clarification session is successful, we process family reunification.

Human sexuality. Oftentimes offenders are sexualized. Both their persona (physiology, mannerisms, clothing, etc.) and their relationships are more sexualized than non-offending peers. It is difficult for them to discuss sexuality and experiences. They believe many myths. It is essential to process fantasies and masturbation.

Relapse prevention. Patients repetitively examine thought patterns. They recognize thinking errors and know their warning signals. Support groups in the community must be available.

Integrating Treatment with a Heterogeneous Milieu

Status in the behavior system. Sexual offender issues, i.e., boundaries, cues to excitement, degrees of independence, and power issues must take precedence over automatic reinforcers in a milieu management system. Statuses or levels of freedom should require sex offender therapist approval.

Experiencing therapeutic home visits. Visits cannot be experienced until it is ascertained that the victim is safe and has made progress in his or her own treatment of being able to say no, and that the sex offender has accomplished completion of phases through clarification with the victim.

Risk management and liability. Admission criteria is critical. Histories of violent sexual offenses, lengthy histories of assaultive behavior even though unrelated to the sexual offense, and I.Q. below 80 need more than a staff secure setting. It is expected patients will replay offending behaviors both analogously, e.g., drawings, fantasies, conversation, and symptomatically, e.g., engagement in behaviors precursory to offending (each offender has an stylized foreplay modus operandi). When such behavior occurs, a well supervised milieu will intervene prior to an offense occurring. This is excellent grist for the therapeutic mill.

When a patient commits an offense which was a presenting problem, e.g., a fondler who successfully fondled the school librarian, that patient must be transferred to a more intensive setting. The victim and family must be acknowledged. Protocols should parallel those implemented for other types of patient endangerment occur with the addition of a sexual abuse component. As of this paper, no patient has completed a violent or penetrative sexual offense. We have reviewed our programs and protocols with our insurer for compliance, and our facility is JCAHO accredited.

Peer relationships. A common denominator is the milieu being restricted to conduct disorders. Traits include violating rights of others, violating norms, aggression, poor self-esteem, vandalism, impulsiveness, irritability, anxiety, depression, under-achievement, and little concern for the wishes, feelings, and well-being of others (American Psychiatric Association, 1987). Such common traits allow common programming for sex offenders and other patients. By treating the sexual offender in a mixed milieu we also give him an opportunity to experience how others perceive him and how to cope. We view our offenders as a subgroup such as those in groups for substance abuse, anger control, etc. The subgroups allow for treatment focus and mutual support.

Some offenders are treated as a whole house issue, e.g., a homosexual fondler who is so clever that the victim doesn't realize the fondling. Some highly persuasive, attractive, or aggressive homosexual offenders need their own rooms.

OUTCOME

Fourteen sexual offenders entered treatment since 1985 and were discharged in 1988 or prior. Of the 14, 4 did not complete treatment. Of the 10 who completed, we were unable to follow up 2. Of the remaining 8, 2 had coping difficulties unrelated to sexual offenses. The remaining 6 have done well as far as we can say. We introduce the caveat, "as far as we can say" because the average sexual offender commits 300 to 600 offenses prior to being arrested. Of the 4 who did not complete the program, 2 are doing well, and 2 are not. None have reoffended as far as we can say. The 12 sexual offenders we have been able to follow up show no evidence of reoffending after two or more years discharge.

DISCUSSION

Some conduct disorders outgrow their symptomatology in adulthood. Sex abuse presents another type of developmental problem. Follow-up is two to five years after treatment, often placing the offender at ages of anywhere from nineteen to twenty-three years of age. Without consistent aftercare (which is not readily available in our society), relapse could occur as new developmental tasks and stress around these tasks, i.e., parenting, evolve. The issue of sexual offending relapse deserves more attention in the literature. Freud's abandoned idea of sexual trauma deserves more consideration.

CONCLUSION

Sexual offender treatment can be efficacious in an open milieu of adolescent male conduct disorders. A mixed milieu poses many therapeutic advantages: perpetrators in the milieu help to raise consciousness of other victims and offenders. A mixed milieu prevents the offender subgroup from developing perpetrator defenses while encouraging therapeutic alliance among the offender subgroup. Sexual offenders can more quickly learn how the non-offending world views them and what they have to do to cope in the non-offending world.

REFERENCES

American Psychiatric Association (1987). *Diagnostic and Statistical Manual of Mental and Nervous Disorders (Third Edition-Revised): DSM-III-R*. Washington, D.C.: The American Psychiatric Association.

Burdsal, C., Force, R., & Klingsporn, M. (1989). Treatment Effectiveness in young male offenders. *Residential Treatment for Children & Youth*, Vol. 7(2), p. 75-88.

Groth, N., & Loredo, C. (1981). Juvenile sexual offenders: Guidelines for Assessment. *International Journal of Offender Therapy and Comparative Criminology*, 25.

Kazdin, Alan E. (1987). *Conduct Disorders in Childhood and Adolescence*. Beverly Hills, California: Sage Publications.

Klingsporn, M., Force, R., & Burdsal, C. (1990). The effectiveness of various degrees and circumstances of program completion of young male offenders in a residential treatment center. *Journal of Clinical Psychology*, Vol. 46, No. 4, pp. 491-500.

The Survivors Project:
A Multimodal Therapy Program
for Adolescents in Residential Treatment
Who Have Survived Child Sexual Abuse

Bruce S. Zahn, MA
Seran E. Schug, MCAT, ADTR

SUMMARY. *The Survivors Project* is a multimodal therapeutic program that addresses the unique attributes and treatment needs of adolescents in residential treatment who have suffered from child sexual abuse. The need for specialized treatment arose from clinical observation that many of the adolescents being referred to our residential treatment center had reported histories of childhood trauma accompanied by symptomatic behaviors and intrapsychic conflicts commonly seen in sexually abused youth. *The Survivors Project* utilizes an integrated therapeutic approach and includes structured group psychotherapy, movement therapy, and psychoeducational stress management training group. This program was designed to facilitate the understanding and working through of powerful post-traumatic seque-

---

This paper is based on a presentation at the 34th Annual Meeting of the American Association of Children's Residential Centers, St. Petersburg Beach, FL, October 10-13, 1990.

The project was supported by an intramural grant from The Devereux Foundation Institute of Clinical Training and Research, Steven I. Pfeiffer, PhD, ABPP, Director.

Mr. Zahn may be written at the Presbyterian Medical Center of Philadelphia, 39th and Market Streets, Philadelphia, PA 19104.

65

lae of child sexual abuse through emotional, cognitive and sensory experiences. This article contains an in-depth examination of clinical case material related to verbal and nonverbal patterns of group process behavior, observed in the *The Survivors Project* groups, as it specifically relates to survivors issues.

INTRODUCTION

The tragedy of child sexual abuse in children and adolescents has grown in astounding numbers in recent years, often with devastating effects upon these young victims. According to recent research, between 150,000 and 200,000 new cases of child sexual abuse are reported each year (Finkelhor and Hotaling, 1984; National Center on Child Abuse and Neglect, 1981). Studies by Browne and Finkelhor (1986) have indicated that severe symptoms have been observed in 46 to 66 percent of sexually abused children. Forty to eighty percent of these symptoms are related to anxiety and its associated manifestations of autonomic hyperarousal, avoidant behaviors, and reexperiencing phenomena (Anderson et al., 1981; DeFrancis, 1969; Tufts, 1984). These symptoms constitute partial criteria for the DSM III-R diagnostic category of post-traumatic stress disorder (PTSD).

A review of the client records at the Devereux Foundation's Gateway Villas Treatment Programs during September, 1989, indicated that at least two-thirds of the adolescent female population identified traumatic sexual abuse as part of their history, even though in each case, the reason for referral to residential treatment did not include emotional or behavioral disturbance directly attributed to abuse. Consequently, the authors felt that it was of critical importance to identify emotional and behavioral sequelae of traumatic sexual abuse as part of the clinical picture in this population, and to develop appropriate treatment strategies.

ISSUES IN RESIDENTIAL TREATMENT

Sexually abused children have been found to exhibit a wide range of symptomatic behaviors and intrapsychic problems. Behavioral symptoms that correspond to post-traumatic symptomatology can include enuresis (Swanson & Biaggio, 1985), sleep disturbances (Berliner & Ernst, 1982; Burgess, Groth, Holstrom & Sgroi, 1978; Mannarino & Cohen, 1986; Shelton, 1963), running away and truancy (Berliner & Ernst, 1982), learning problems (Bender & Blau, 1937; Burgess, Hartman, McClausland & Powers, 1984; Kaufman, Peck & Taguri, 1954; Seidner & Calhoun, 1984), hyperactivity (Bender & Blau, 1937), and inappropriate sexual behavior (Kaufman et al., 1954; Mannarino & Cohen, 1986). Intrapsychic problems can include depression, anxiety, and suicidal ideation (Bagley & Ramsey, 1985; Berliner & Ernst, 1982; Kaufman et al., 1954; Rist, 1979; Sedney & Brooks, 1984; Briere & Runtz, 1985). Sexually abused children also appear to have difficulty in interpersonal relationships (Bender & Grugett, 1951; Berliner & Ernst, 1982; Burgess, Groth & McClausland, 1981; Courtois, 1979; Mannarino & Cohen, 1986; Tong, Oates & McDowell, 1987). Several researchers have found links between sexual abuse and more serious problems such as psychosis (Swanson, 1985) and multiple personality (Coons, 1986).

The overwhelming effects of traumatic life events that overpower the human coping response were identified by the American Psychiatric Association in DSM III (APA, 1980) by creation of the diagnostic category, Post-Traumatic Stress Disorder. In many cases, the diagnosis of PTSD has been reserved for adult veterans of war or victims of natural disasters or terroristic threats. Current discussions among top researchers in the area of psychological trauma have left the issue of whether or not PTSD is a diagnosable disorder in children and adolescents unresolved. Nevertheless, many clinicians who have worked with child and adolescent survivors of sexual abuse acknowledge the presence of post-traumatic sequelae such as hyperarousal, memory impairment and distortion, depression and impaired coping responses (Burgess and Holstrom, 1979; Van der Kolk, 1988; Emery and Smith, 1987; Gil, 1987; Sgroi, 1982).

One distressing finding in the recent literature (Doyle and Bauer, 1989) is that many of the emotionally disturbed youth who are referred for treatment to residential programs have been subjected to physical, psychological, and/or sexual abuse, yet are not identified as such by mental health professionals and are not formally diagnosed as suffering from the constellation of symptoms that hallmark the sequelae of abuse.

Identification of the constellation of symptoms associated with traumatic abuse is essential if treatment is to be effective (Hyman, Zelikoff, & Clarke, 1988). For example, a client, Pat (not her real name), a victim of repetitive, unpredictable physical and sexual abuse by several members of her family, had been in psychiatric treatment facilities for over seven years, yet had not been treated for the sequelae of sexual abuse. Instead, her maladjusted behavior had been interpreted as being organically/neurologically based, and her repetitive self-destructive acting out was interpreted as being a manifestation of organically-driven perseveration.

Another interpretation of Pat's symptoms seems plausible. According to traumagenic theory, survivors of traumatic sexual abuse may repeat or reenact the abusive acts as a means of attempting mastery of the overwhelming conflict (Burgess & Hartman, 1988). This is called "reenactment" of the trauma. According to this theory, traumatic memory remains active and unprocessed until such time as it can be therapeutically "worked through" and placed into past memory. Behaviors that look "perseverative" may actually be behaviors that are repetitions of the response to trauma which have not yet been processed. Within this model, we might view Pat's reenactment behavior as being symptomatic of the unresolved traumatic effects of sexual abuse.

In residential treatment, reenactment may also be observed in acting out of power struggles with staff and peers, and in eliciting negative and punitive responses from staff. Sexual abuse is an issue of "power," not only "sexual desire" (Sgroi, 1982). The relationship between victim and victimizer is symbolic of power issues, sometimes with sexualized behavior being of secondary consequence. In the victim role, the message given to the child is one of powerlessness and lack of control, which becomes internalized and intractable. In reenactment or mastery play, the youngster may alternate between victim and victimizer roles which can be observed in the treatment milieu. Self-abusive and aggressive behaviors may also be a manifestation of reenactment and an attempt for mastery over the trauma, when viewed from this perspective.

Another client, Diane (not her real name), had been in residential schools for five years after ongoing conflicts with her adoptive family members. Diane was removed from her natural family due to neglect, incest, and extrafamilial sexual abuse. Problematic behaviors such as promiscuity, excessive demandingness toward adults, lack of trust, secrecy, pseudoindependence, manipulation and rebelliousness in pre-pubertal years, continued to be observed years later in residential treatment. In addition, Diane was diagnosed as suffering from a severe learning disability, with expressive and receptive language deficits, which was used to explain her inability to process verbally presented information and utilize verbal means of self-expression.

Another interpretation of these behaviors could be that Diane was struggling to cope with her unresolved thoughts and feelings regarding the trauma, and her acting out symptoms could be understood within the context of trauma theory. For example, the excessive demanding quality of her interactions with staff, and her fears of not being protected by them, which frustrated some staff and overly engaged others, was seen as a manifestation of perceptions and feelings related to helplessness and vulnerability. Once Diane began to connect her feelings, thoughts and behaviors (to a lesser degree) to the abuse, she was able to correct her perceptions and less frequently interpret milieu experiences as being potentially abusive.

In view of the active nature of her power struggles, Diane did not seem to have enough conflict-free ego resources at her disposal to process neutral information and thus manifested language deficits. Once she became more trusting of others, she found it easier to put her thoughts and feelings into words. Within one year, her special education teacher noted that Diane's achievement score improved by three grade levels.

Another phenomenon observed in the residential treatment of sexual abuse survivors is the spontaneous affiliation with similar peers through symbolic activity. As clinicians, we observed milieu group behavior which appeared to express the clients' underlying needs to play out various roles within the sexual abuse situation such as victim, perpetrator, rescuer, witness, and inciter. Prior to any formalized treatment intervention of these issues, staff had observed that a small group of these clients appeared to have developed an informal group system in order to play out their conflicts related to these roles.

Consequently, we saw the need to formalize a group treatment program that would address trauma-related issues within a structured therapeutic framework.

TREATMENT CONSIDERATIONS AND MODALITIES

Most researchers and clinicians agree that the basic treatment process in helping survivors of child sexual abuse to recover involves at least four major categories: (1) *communication,* in which the client learns how to identify and express complex feelings, (2) *sorting out,* in which she[1] explores an understanding of what happened during the trauma, (3) *education,* in which the client learns to understand the specific elements of the traumatizing experience, and (4) *perspective,* in which the client's experience is accepted as something that has happened to her without the need for exaggeration and minimization of its impact (James, 1989).

There are four major steps that are generally recognized as facilitating youngsters being able to integrate traumatizing experiences, consisting of: (1) clarifying why it is necessary to slowly and carefully examine what happened, (2) helping to re-create the traumatic events in play and fantasy, in which the clients can be victorious survivors rather than victims, (3) enabling the youngsters to acknowledge their own ideas, feelings, and behaviors related to the traumatic event, (4) assisting them in accepting the realities of their experience without minimizing or exaggerating the significance of what happened, thus helping these clients to experience mastery (James, 1989).

Emery and Smith (1987) argued that stress disorders are only one component of the entire trauma complex, the primary consequence of which is the individual's proclivity to reenact the circumstances

---

1. The authors have chosen to use the pronoun "she" to refer to the survivor of sexual abuse with full recognition of the existence of both male and female survivors.

that led to victimization. Doyle and Bauer (1989) adapted Emery and Smith's observations into a Seven Treatment Objective Recovery Model that included the following components: (1) establishment of a therapeutic relationship, (2) education on the stress recovery process, (3) management and reduction of stress, (4) articulation of affect, (5) reexperience of the trauma, (6) cognitive transformation, and (7) integration of the experience.

Structured group therapy has been a core treatment modality that has been discussed in the literature as well. Sturkie (1983) outlined the following themes, among others, that might be addressed in such a group for survivors of traumatic sexual abuse: believability, guilt and responsibility, body integrity, secrecy and sharing, anger, powerlessness, and other life crises.

Creative Arts has also been considered to be an effective component in the treatment of stress and trauma disorders. In 1978, a report by the White House Commission on Mental Health stated that the therapeutic arts must be made available to these youngsters in order to facilitate coping skills in the face of life-threatening traumas. The arts as therapeutic modalities are noted (Sgroi, 1982) to provide individuals with an experience in which rehearsal and mastery over feelings of powerlessness can occur.

THE SURVIVORS PROJECT

The use of a multimodal therapy program, consisting of a structured process group, psychoeducational stress management group, movement therapy, and individual psychotherapy, was designed to help a group of adolescent females who have suffered from child sexual abuse and post-traumatic symptomatology begin to confront and cope with the traumatic effects of abuse.

Trauma assaults the child physically, cognitively, emotionally and spiritually. Because trauma therapy requires a variety of therapeutic tasks in order to achieve mastery and healing (i.e., information processing, relaxation training, education, bonding), treatment strategies and clinical intervention should not be confined to just one area or modality (see Table 1). A child may be able to reach a cognitive understanding of the trauma and know that the event was not her fault; but unless therapeutic work is directed toward irrational thoughts, associated feelings of guilt and anger related to the abuse, or experience of extreme body vulnerability and spiritual confusion, she may not experience relief and may not be able to fully master the traumatic event. It is equally true that if the youngster works through her emotional conflicts and sensory responses but is unable to reach a cognitive understanding of the event, the traumatic experience will not be fully integrated. Moreover, it is our belief that the treatment should include education and skill-building regarding the recovery process in order to help these youngsters to develop the ego strength necessary to maximize their use of the psychotherapy process. Consequently, the multidimensional strategies are often recommended in the treatment of child sexual abuse (Trepper, 1989; James, 1989).

Description of Interventions

The Survivors Project was implemented during eight consecutive weeks. The interventions that comprised *The Survivors Project* were:

A. Structured Process Group
B. Stress Skills Training Group
C. Movement Therapy Group
D. Individual Psychotherapy

The Therapists

The therapists for *The Survivors Project* consisted of a male licensed psychologist and a female registered dance/movement therapist. The therapists had extensive experience in residential treatment of exceptional youth and served as consultants to the entire milieu regarding treatment issues and progress of the members of *The Survivors Project*.

Table 1

TREATMENT MODALITY TREATMENT OBJECTIVES	Structured Process Group	Movement Therapy	Stress Skills Training
Establish Therapeutic Relationship and Group Cohesion	- establishment of group structure - validation of experience of sexual abuse	- establishment of nonverbal interactional synchrony	- establishment of group structure - "anchor for safety" - acknowledgement that stress is universal
Re-education and Relabeling of the Traumatic Experience	- distinguish between guilt and responsibility - differentiation of issues of power, authority and sexuality	- differentiation and substitution of adaptive associations to sensory experiences	- education on the stress recovery process
Enhancement of Coping Skills	- honor survivor skills and encourage generalization of effective survivor skills	- assertion of personal space and personal body boundaries	- teaching relaxation, self-regulation and cognitive coping skills
Acknowledgement of Genuine Feelings & Articulation of Affect	- making anger "safe" - sharing universal feelings of loss, sadness and remorse	- learning body awareness and relaxation exercises - enhancing dynamic quality of expressive movement	- identification of stressors and stress-related responses, followed by implementation of coping skills
Gaining Mastery of the Trauma through Experience	- role play and modelling of adaptive coping responses and techniques	- symbolic play and dance	- graded exposure to stressors - implementation of coping responses
Cognitive Transformation	- development of insight - processing of stored memory - accurate perception of new experiences	- enhanced awareness and understanding of nonverbal cues and nonverbal behavior - neutralization of casual physical contact	- replace maladaptive responses to stressors - utilize variety of effective responses to stressors
Integration of the Experience	- physical, cognitive and emotional unity	- physical, cognitive and emotional unity	- physical, cognitive and emotional unity

The interaction between the particular skills, training, and professional experience of the co-therapists enhanced clients' learning on many different levels, i.e., nonverbal communication styles, modes of thinking and perceiving, and affective response patterns. The advantage of having a male and female co-therapist was to allow the participants to project perceptions about male and female roles and differentiate their feelings toward male and female caretakers. This helped to facilitate a reeducation and relearning of healthy adult sex roles.

In working with adolescent survivors of child sexual abuse, we believe that therapists need to be able to take on various roles such as nurturer, leader, limit-setter and protector, depending upon the needs of the situation. The therapists should develop a level of comfort with issues of anger, hurt, and horror, as these affects are bound to arise in the sessions. We also believe that a mutually supportive relationship between co-therapists is essential in facilitating the therapeutic process and creating a healthy and supportive group milieu.

Client Selection

The participants in *The Survivors Project* consisted of 5 female clients in residential treatment for academic, emotional, and behavioral problems. They were included in the project based upon a documented and substantiated history of traumatic child or early adolescent sexual abuse, documented family acknowledgement of the abuse, voluntary consent and, if under 18 years of age, parental/ guardian consent, and clinical team assessment of ability to profit from an intensive, structured therapeutic program. These criteria necessarily excluded some of our clients who did not have a substantiated history of abuse or who were not assessed to be emotionally stable enough to profit from the interventions. Clients who had a history of child or early adolescent sexual abuse and who were not selected to participate in the project continued with their current treatment program.

The Survivors Project was formally presented to the clinical team, and referrals were generated by individual therapists after discussing the project with their clients who were potential participants. Clients who were referred for participation in the project were then informed of the referral by the co-therapists, who met with each candidate and invited their participation. During this meeting, informed consent was obtained and the program goals and interventions were reviewed.

GROUP INTERVENTION AND RESULTS

Structured Process Group

The design of the Structured Process Group was based on a model that was developed in 1980 at the Pulaski County Child Sexual Abuse Treatment Project located in Little Rock, Arkansas. The group met for eight sessions, and each session dealt with a theme that is particularly relevant to sexually abused adolescents. The goals of the group were:

a. *Validation of the experience:* The therapists acknowledged what happened to the youngsters as being real, and communicated that it was important for each client to understand how the abuse had effected them. We believe that this process was reassuring to their inner experience, which was often denied or unexpressed, i.e., "They know, they believe, they care."

b. *Facilitation of integration process* (i.e., true and connected perception of the event): The therapists attempted to provide a safe and structured environment for thinking about the trauma in a realistic and focused manner.

c. *Provide a container and focus for feelings:* The clients utilized the group structure as an ego support in order to decrease the likelihood of acting out by means of unhealthy behaviors.

d. *Develop coping skills and positive attributional beliefs:* Through teaching, modeling and role-playing, the group members were given opportunities to learn, practice and develop confidence in their ability to actively utilize coping skills as substitutes for previous maladaptive responses to stress (i.e., inaction, withdrawal, aggression).

Seven survivors themes were addressed in the structured process group, with a final session devoted to an integration and summary of the previous work in the group. The themes were addressed in the following order: believability, guilt and responsibility, secrecy and sharing, anger, body integrity and protection, powerlessness, and other life crises.

In order to establish trust within a short-term group, the therapists needed to be highly active in facilitating a safe and supportive milieu. In the initial sessions, the group members displayed attitudes and feelings reflecting ambivalence about participating in open group discussions about their sexual abuse. Consequently, the co-therapists structured and organized tasks related to each theme. For example, in order to facilitate a group discussion about the theme of "guilt and responsibility," a short story about a man who enticed children to touch him for tangible rewards was presented to the group. The clients found it easier to discuss a hypothetical situation, and also used this as a stimulus for relating their own experiences. Understanding motivations and dilemmas for the characters in the story provided the group members with some insight into their own experiences and how they might cope in the future. Similarly, a game was developed by the co-therapists regarding "sharing and secrecy." Group members were asked to write on a piece of blank paper a secret that they would like to share with the group. On another piece of paper, each group member was asked to write a secret that she wished to keep to herself, in order to reinforce appropriate boundaries. The secrets to be shared were revealed within dyads, and reciprocal feelings were elicited. This served to demonstrate to each member that although they could keep some secrets, others could be shared with peers and trusting adults.

Group Process Phenomena

Several interesting phenomena emerged during the eight weeks of the Structured Process Group. As the co-therapists, we observed that different roles within the group process took on unique characteristics based upon survivor issues. Bion's (1959) model of group process served as theoretical framework to understand roles. We labelled the roles as *Avoider/Denier, Needy Doubter, Voyeur/Witness, Obeyer/Follower,* and *Conflicted Emoter.* These roles were consistent within group members across the various group interventions.

The *Avoider/Denier* participated in the groups by physically and psychologically distancing, and actively denying that sexual assault had a significant impact on her life. She also attempted to distract the group from the tasks. The co-therapists recognized that survivors sometimes try to cope with their trauma by denying the existence of the traumatic event or denying its effects. By identifying for this client her need to defend against overwhelming thoughts and affects, the co-therapists facilitated her participation in the group and encouraged her to come to grips with the reality that the abuse had occurred.

The *Needy Doubter* expressed ambivalence regarding her need to be believed, nurtured and protected. Her need to avoid seemed to stem from fear of rejection and abandonment. She initially aligned with the *Avoider/Denier*, yet periodically engaged in therapeutic tasks, demonstrating attunement with the co-therapists. By the end of the eight weeks, she had formed a positive therapeutic relationship with the co-therapists. Her need for adult caretakers to protect her and attend to her predominated over needs for peer affiliation. As long as the co-therapists concretely communicated that they were respectful and attentive to her needs, she engaged in the group process and began to work on survivors issues.

The *Voyeur/Witness* passively participated in the groups and appeared to be withholding information about her past experiences and related feelings. Nonetheless, she was an integral part of the group, and it was clear to group members that she was observing the events in the group. The co-therapists recognized this behavior as possibly corresponding to a dissociative defense against overwhelming stimuli. The literature on sexual abuse often describes circumstances in which survivors discuss their experiences as if they were "watching" the event from a distance (James, 1989). Similarly, this client needed to psychologically distance herself by physically shutting down, i.e., lying on a mat with her head down, with passive weight, but keeping visually and auditorially in touch with the group activities. The co-therapists consistently acknowledged that they were aware that this client was, in fact, participating in the group process. A voyeuristic quality to this client's behavior was also noted, as she appeared to derive satisfaction from the others sharing their emotional experiences. Consultation with her individual therapist revealed that this client became highly active in working on survivors issues in individual psychotherapy, despite her continued passivity in the group sessions, implying that she was processing the feelings at some level.

The *Obeyer/Follower* acted mostly as a task leader in the group process. She was considered to be an individual who could intellectually acknowledge the effects of her abuse, but who had not yet integrated her affect with cognition. Obeyance, although it appeared to facilitate task completion, was identified as a crucial survivors issue, in that there was a quality of "let's get this over with," which is a common experience in survivors of sexual abuse. This attitude and behavior needed to be identified by the co-therapists so as not to be misled into believing that the *Obeyer/Follower* was as integrated as she might otherwise appear. Accordingly, our intervention was to help this client use the defense of "compliance" with a more self-assertive quality. For example, the therapist might state, "Thank you for *deciding* to lead the discussion today."

The *Conflicted Emoter* was seen as an emotional leader who, at times, wished to escape from the group process. She openly expressed the group's anger, fear, sadness and vulnerability, yet clearly felt uncomfortable in doing so. At times, she projected that she was compelled to act out these emotions for the group, and she expressed urges to retreat from these feelings. As co-therapists, we felt that it was important to support the *Conflicted Emoter's* need for clear interpersonal boundaries. She was in touch with her feelings, but she was unable to cognitively connect them to their source, resulting in a lack of integration between cognition and affect. Containment of affect was important for her until such time that she and the group were able to own, modulate, and integrate the expression of affect.

Transference and Countertransference

In the group process, issues of transference and countertransference will naturally evolve and need to be addressed. The manifestation of transference and countertransference in *The Survivors Project* groups seemed to be related to overarching survivors themes.

Projected affect may often elicit strong countertransference feelings of anger, disregard, and hurt. As co-therapists, we found it to be beneficial to identify and work through these feelings outside of the group sessions. It is our belief that this helped us to create a safe milieu in which the survivors could direct their anger and fear.

One of our most striking observations was that many intense feelings were projected onto the male co-therapist, which needed to be absorbed rather than directly confronted. Confrontation might be perceived as being too intrusive and threatening to their safety. For example, the *Conflicted Emoter* consistently projected her fears of literally being looked at as a sexual object by the male co-therapist and she demanded, "Stop looking at me." The male co-therapist helped to create a feeling of safety by differentiating between objective reality and psychological reality, acknowledging her fear, and respecting her need to avoid eye contact. After five weeks, this client was able to tolerate periodic eye contact and she was able to interact and share feelings with the male co-therapist.

An attempt to engage the female co-therapist in directing anger toward the male co-therapist was enacted by the group members. The anger from the clients was so strong it was, at times, tempting to identify with these feelings. However, it was important to accept and support the clients' self-expression without identifying with their feelings. The female therapist, as protector and nurturer, was available to confront the projections onto the male co-therapist through corrective feedback. One form of confrontation that was used consisted of teaching skills for being able to differentiate sexual and neutral nonverbal behavior.

As transference and countertransference issues were able to be worked through, the co-therapists were more free to interchange roles of nurturer/protector and task leader or limit setter. This facilitated therapeutic growth toward being able to perceive adults in alternate roles and to improve the quality of interactional behavior with adult caretakers in the residential setting.

Movement Therapy

To fully heal from the trauma of sexual abuse, expression and integration must occur both verbally and non-verbally, i.e., through words and body movement. Since sexual abuse is experienced both physically and emotionally, it is our belief that treatment should include an approach that intervenes in these modalities.

> . . .The body never forgets. Although the mind may deny the invasion, the bodily responses are ever present and affect the victim's life in ways often incomprehensible to others. (Vassington, in Sgroi, 1988)

The movement therapy segment of this program was structured to address the various problems that are manifest in or derived from the body experience. One of the most significant responses to abuse is the development of a poor body image. Since survivors of sexual abuse had to endure assaults to the body which were experienced as forced and unpleasant, they often develop a disgust or dislike for their own body, its' appearance and its' functioning. This has comprehensive repercussions due to the notion that body image is a primary experience of the sense of self (Lowen, 1958). Emotional disturbances may also result in part from harmful experiences to the body (Fisher & Cleveland, 1978). This refers to body boundary and body perception disturbances which impair reality testing and impaired body image.

Creative arts therapies including movement therapy may also more directly access those traumatic memories which are stored symbolically through various sensory images, and often difficult to verbally express (Sgroi, 1982; James, 1989; Johnson, 1987). For example, the movement therapist worked with a client who began to shake and physically retreat from her when the therapist smiled. By mirroring this to the client, she learned that the perpetrator of this client's abuse often smiled before assaulting this young girl. By making this connection for the client, allowing unlinking of the association between smiling and the onset of abuse, new connections and more adaptive associations to the smiling facial expression could be accomplished.

Another client did not verbally express any anger or anxiety about being sexually abused following abandonment by her mother. However, during improvisational play with props, which occurred in the context of movement therapy, she would name a beach ball a "baby" and kick it and throw it in the closet.

Nonverbal play may highlight the creative ways with which these youth were able to defend against the overwhelming internal and external stimuli of the abuse. For example, one client expressed her defensive posture when she and the movement therapist were engaged in tossing an imaginary ball. The movement therapist asked her to "keep" the ball, yet she symbolically split it into two pieces stating, "It's too much to hold it in one piece. I have to separate it into pieces, then I can keep it." This may be thought of as an example of the defenses of compartmentalization and dissociation of feelings. These defenses were confronted through nonverbal play, such as helping the client to take the broken pieces of the imaginary ball and, together with the movement therapist, hold them in one piece. When the client was ready, she was able to hold the ball on her own, thus symbolizing the ability to contain many different feelings at once.

Case studies indicate that during their early abuse, survivors were often given conflicting or ambiguous nonverbal cues before being subjected to the abuse. This experience may confuse survivors with regard to reading others' more culturally common nonverbal behavior. Survivors of sexual abuse also often show patterns of non-verbal behavior which predispose them to being revictimized (Goodill, 1987); as stated earlier, the survivor may attempt to reenact the traumatic event in order to master the conflicts and feelings associated with the event. This reenactment is unconscious, and thus the behavioral patterns developed in the "repetition compulsion" become characteristic of their interactional repertoire. For example, a client working in movement therapy did not understand why, during leisure activities in the residential unit, a male peer was touching her breast. When asked to role play the situation with the movement therapist by sitting in relation to the therapist where she was sitting in relation to the boy, this client surprisingly moved to sit on the therapist's lap. The client confided that she did not understand that this behavior could be construed as being provocative.

To address these problems, participants in *The Survivors Project* received group movement therapy one time per week for the duration of the eight weeks. The movement therapist attempted to establish and support group cohesion by encouraging movement dynamics which are reflective of reciprocity, rapport, attunement and trust. Interactional synchrony, expressed by moving to a similar rhythm, spatial orientation, and quality, typically facilitates a group unity (Kestenberg, 1975; Condon, 1968; Stern, 1985; Chapple, 1970). The movement therapist actively organized synchronous experiences, by establishing a rhythmic movement for the group to follow, or using a prop, such as a stretch cloth, which spatially organized the group.

Movement therapy provided an alternative mode of communication through which the clients could progressively express and work through anxiety-producing experiences. Structured dance improvisation and improvisational play with props set the stage for creative, spontaneous, yet controlled expression of images, feelings or stories. The clients were initially limited in their expression affect in an organized and dramatic manner. The movement therapist took an active role in teaching them the different qualities of movement that may represent different feeling states, i.e., strength directed in a downward motion was viewed as "anger" and light, delicate movement was seen as "feeling good." The clients eventually learned to look at others' movement and label the feelings that they felt while observing movements, as well as the feelings they thought the mover was experiencing.

A central aim of the movement therapy group was to provide ego support to the clients through non-verbal means. Enabling abused individuals to define their own personal space and exercise control over that space has been shown to help them regain a sense of control and ownership over their bodies and thus, over their lives (Goodill, 1987). Games in which the clients practiced being approached and setting interpersonal boundaries appeared to foster a sense of power and enjoyment. During one session, clients shared experiences in which they had said "no" and asserted themselves with others.

The movement therapy group was mostly directed toward helping the clients to explore and identify attitudes toward their own bodies and begin to construct a more positive body image. Accepting and reflecting the client's initiations in movement increased awareness of how they presented themselves to the world and in turn, aided in empowering them to intentionally design and assert a new communicative style to the world.

Honoring and enhancing those aspects which contributed to the clients' survival was also a significant part of the treatment. For example, a passive avoidant style, exhibited through passive movement qualities, was mirrored by the therapist with a transformation of passivity to a relaxed movement quality, thus making this survival skill generalizable and more adaptive. An aggressive stance was modified with an attempt to develop self-assertion skills (i.e., use of strong downward rather than attacking type movements).

Thus, the clients were given a new non-verbal expressive "vocabulary" that was coherent, organized and personally fulfilling.

The process of accepting and integrating the memories, sensations and emotional upheaval of the sexual abuse was acknowledged as being difficult. In body terms, through becoming more sensitive and discriminative of body sensations and physical reactions to various stimuli, confusion decreased and clarity of feelings emerged. Breathing and relaxation exercises allowed the clients to experience affect and sensation in a pleasant and nonthreatening setting. Accordingly, defenses of numbing or experiences of hyperarousal could begin to be replaced by full, yet controlled experience of affect.

Finally, movement therapy provided a nurturing experience so that the clients could enjoy physical contact in a positive, supportive and non-sexual context. Neutralization of kinesthetic stimulation was accomplished by unlinking associations of touch and abuse, and by developing skills to differentiate between neutral and sexual stimulation. This was accomplished by performing age-appropriate dance games in which the clients were gradually exposed to neutralized tactile experiences, until they became comfortable enough to initiate nurturing touch with the therapist, i.e., hugs or hand shakes.

Stress Skills Training

This in-depth training introduced the clients to the skills they need to handle stress in their lives. The curriculum portion of the training was adapted by the co-therapists to teach a holistic approach to stress. The curriculum was designed to help participants to: understand the nature of stress; analyze its sources; use a variety of approaches to handling stressful situations; identify resources for coping, and design personal action plans (Tubesing, 1979).

Burgess (1990) has emphasized the need to help survivors of sexual trauma to be able to manage arousal reactions which may represent a reexperience of the original trauma. Through structured practice of controlled arousal, the youngsters were able to take the primary steps of engaging in trauma therapy. The stress skills group also provided a forum in which the co-therapists could actively be nurturing and supportive of the clients. This group served as an "anchor of safety" for the other component groups in *The Survivors Project*.

CONCLUSIONS

The Survivors Project was a multimodal pilot program designed to augment the individual treatment of adolescent survivors of child sexual abuse in residential treatment. The strength of a multimodal treatment approach is the fostering of the integration of sensory, perceptual and cognitive experiences for the survivor who does, in fact, encounter the traumatic events on all of these levels. An additional benefit of the project was to facilitate reconceptualization of problematic behaviors in order to develop more effective methods of client management in the milieu.

The reality of working in an open residential setting imposed natural constraints on the timing and depth of the therapeutic work that could be accomplished. Due to the short-term nature of the project, issues of anchoring for safety, learning coping skills, developing self-regulation, and setting personal boundaries were given primary attention.

Because *The Survivors Project* was implemented in a residential treatment setting, the co-therapists viewed communication within the milieu as being of fundamental value. Issues of transference and countertransference were so strong that milieu staff needed to have a heightened sensitivity and awareness of the specific issues of survivors of sexual abuse, especially when they relate to issues of power. We believe that the recognition that sexual abuse is an abuse of power and a betrayal of adult responsibility, would help the treatment team members to react to the "acting out" behaviors of survivors in a more therapeutic manner. We also believe that in-servicing by trained staff and consultants, and conducting team meetings where open discussions of transference and countertransference issues occurred, can help to ensure the identification and appropriate treatment of post-traumatic symptomatology in survivors of child sexual abuse.

BIBLIOGRAPHY

Anderson, S.C., Bach, C.M., and Griffith, S. (1981). Psychosexual sequelae in interfamilial victims of sexual assault and abuse. Paper presented at the Third International Conference on Child Abuse and Neglect, Amsterdam, The Netherlands.

Bagley, C. & Ramsey, R. (1985). Disrupted childhood and vulnerability to sexual assault: Long-term sequels with implications for counseling. Paper presented at the Conference on Counseling the Sexual Abuse Survivor. Winnepeg, Canada.

Bartenieff, I. & Lewis, D. (1980). *Body movement: Coping with the environment.* NY: Gordon & Breach Science Publishers.

Bass, E. & Davis, L. (1988). *The Courage to heal: A guide for women survivors of child sexual abuse.* New York: Harper and Row.

Bender, L. & Blau, A. (1937). The reaction of children to sexual relation with adults. *American Journal of Orthopsychiatry, 17,* 500-518.

Bender, L. & Grugett, A.E. (1952). A followup report on children who had atypical sexual experience. *American Journal of Orthopsychiatry, 17,* 500-518.

Bentovim, A. (1987). The diagnosis of child sexual abuse. *Bulletin of the Royal College of Psychiatrist, 11,* 295-299.

Berliner, L. & Ernst, E. (1982). Group work with pre-adolescent sexual assault victims. In Irving Stuart & Joanne Greer (Eds.), *Victims of sexual aggression: Men, women, children,* New York: Van Nostrand Reingold Co.

Berman, P. (1990). Group therapy techniques for sexually abused preteen girls. *Child Welfare, LXIX* (3), 239-252.

Briere, J. (1984). The effects of childhood sexual abuse on later psychological functioning: Defining a "post-sexual abuse syndrome." Paper presented at the Third National Conference on Sexual Victimization of Children, Washington, D.C.

Browne, A. & Finkelhor, D. (1986). Impact of child sexual abuse: A review of the research. *Psychological Bulletin,* 99 66-77.

Burgess, A.W. (1990). Child trauma: Sexual victimization. Paper presented at the Horsham Foundation, Horsham, PA. May 10, 1990.

Burgess, A. & Groth, N. (October, 1980). Child sexual abuse. Keynote speech presented at the Third National Symposium on Violence in Families, Hot Springs, Arkansas.

Burgess, A.W. & Holstrom, L.L. (1979). *Rape: Crisis and recovery.* Bowie, MD: Robert S. Brady.

Burgess, A.W., Groth, N., Holstrom, L. & Sgroi, S. (1978). *Sexual assault of children and adolescents.* Lexington, Mass.: D.C. Heath and Co.

Burgess, A. W., Groth, N., & McClausland, M.P. (1981). Child sex initiation rings. *American Journal of Orthopsychiatry, 51,* 110-119.

Burgess, A.W., Hartman, C.R., McClausland, M.P. & Powers, P. (1984). Response patterns in children and adolescents exploited through sex rings and pornography. *American Journal of Psychiatry, 141,* 378-383.

Carozza, P.M. & Hiersteiner, C.L. (1983). Young female incest victims in treatment: Stages of growth seen with a group art therapy model. *Clinical Social Work Journal, 10*(3), 165-173.

Chapple, E. (1970). *Cultural and biological man. Explorations in behavioral anthropology.* Ithaca, NY: Holt, Rinehart & Winston, Inc.

Christup, H. (1978). The effect of dance therapy on the concept of body image. In M.N. Costonis (Ed.), *Therapy in motion,* Chicago: University of Illinois Press.

Chu, J. (1988). Ten traps for therapists in the treatment of trauma survivors. *Dissociation, 1*, (4), 24-32.

Condon,W.S. (1968). Linguistic-kinesic research and dance therapy. American Dance Therapy Proceedings, Third Annual Conference, 21-44.

Coons, P.M. (1986). Child abuse and multiple personality disorder: Review of the literature and suggestions for treatment. *Child Abuse and Neglect, 10,* 455-462.

Diagnostic and statistical manual of mental disorders, Third Edition Revised. (1988). American Psychiatric Association, Washington, D.C.

DeFrancis, V. (1969). *Protecting the child victim of sex crimes committed by adults.* Denver, Colo.: American Humane Association.

Doyle, J.S. & Bauer, S.K. (1989). Post-traumatic stress disorder in children: Its identification and treatment in a residential setting for emotionally disturbed youth. *Journal of Traumatic Stress, 2*(3), 275-288.

Emery, P., & Smith, J. (1987). *The treatment of post-traumatic stress disorder based on ten propositions.*

Eth, S. & Pynoos, R. (Eds.) (1985). *Post-traumatic stress disorder in children.* Washington, D.C. American Psychiatric Press.

Finkelhor, D. & Browne, A. (1985). The traumatic impact of child sexual abuse: A conceptualization. *American Journal of Orthopsychiatry, 55*(4), 530-541.

Finkelhor, D. & Hotaling, G.T. (1984). Sexual abuse in a national incidence study of child abuse and neglect: An appraisal. *Child Abuse and Neglect, 8,* 23-32.

Fisher, S. & Cleveland, S. (1978). Personality, body perception and body image boundary. In M.N. Costonis (Ed.), *Therapy in motion.* Chicago, IL: University of Illinois Press.

Foa, E. (1990). Post-traumatic stress disorder. Presentation at the meeting of the Philadelphia Behavior Therapy Association, Philadelphia, PA, March 8, 1990.

Gil, E. (1987). *Treatment approaches with survivors of childhood abuse.* Walnut Creek, CA: Launch Press.

Goodill, S.W. (1987). Dance/movement therapy with abused children. *The Arts in Psychotherapy, 14,* 59-68.

Goodwin, J. (1988). Post-traumatic symptoms in abused children. *Journal of Traumatic Stress, 1*(4), 475-488.

Hartman, C.R. & Burgess, A.W. (1988). Information processing of trauma: Case application of a model. *Journal of Interpersonal Violence, 3*(4), 443-457.

Hyman, I.A., Zelikoff, W., & Clarke, J. (1988). Psychological and physical abuse in schools: A paradigm for understanding posttraumatic stress in children. *Journal of Traumatic Stress, 1*(2), 243-267.

James, B. (1989). *Treating traumatized children: New insights and creative interventions.* Lexington, MA: Lexington Books.

Johnson, D.R. (1987). The role of the creative arts therapies in the diagnosis and treatment of psychological trauma. *The Arts in Psychotherapy, 14,* 7-13.

Kaslow, N. & Eicher, V. (1988). Body image therapy: A combined creative arts therapy and verbal psychotherapy approach. *The Arts in Psychotherapy, 15,* 177-188.

Kaufman, I., Peck, A., & Taguri, C. (1954). The family constellation and overt incestuous relations between father and daughter. *American Journal of Orthopsychiatry, 24,* 266-279.

Keane, T.M. & Kaloupek, D.G. (1982). Imaginal flooding in the treatment of post-traumatic stress disorder. *Journal of Consulting and Clinical Psychology, 50,* 138-140.

Kestenberg, J. (1975). *Children and parents: Psychoanalytic studies in development.* New York: Jason Aronson.

Kilpatrick, D.G., Veronen, L.J., & Resic, P.A. (1982). Psychological sequelae to rape: Assessment and treatment strategies. In D.M. Doleys, R.L. Meredith, & A.R. Ciminero (Eds.), *Behavioral medicine: Assessment and treatment strategies.* New York: Plenum.

Knittie, B.J. & Tuana, S.J. (1980). Group therapy as primary treatment for adolescent victims of intrafamilial sexual abuse. *Clinical Social Work Journal, 8*(4), 236-242.

Lowen, A. (1958). *Physical dynamics of character structure: Bodily form and movement in analytic therapy.* NY: Grune and Stratton, Inc.

Mannarino, A.P. & Cohen, J.A. (1986). A clinical demographic study of sexually abused children. *Child Abuse and Neglect, 10,* 17-23.

McElroy, L.P. & McElroy, R.A. (1989). Psychoanalytically oriented psychotherapy with sexually abused children. *Journal of Mental Health Counseling, 11*(3), 244-258.

National Center on Child Abuse and Neglect (1981). Study findings: National study on the incidence and severity of child abuse and neglect (DHHS Pub. No. (OHDS) 81-30325). Washington, D.C.: U.S. Government Printing Office.

Rist, K. (1979). Incest: Theoretical and clinical views. *American Journal of Orthopsychiatry, 56,* 680-690.

Schmais, C. (1985). Healing processes in group dance therapy. *American Journal of Dance Therapy, 8,* 17-36.

Sedney, M.A. & Brooks, B. (1984). Factors associated with a history of childhood sexual experience in a nonclinical female population. *Journal of the American Academy of Child Psychiatry, 23,* 215-218.

Seidner, A. & Calhoun, K.S. (1984). Childhood sexual abuse: Factors related to differential adjustment. Paper presented at the 2nd Annual National Family and Violence Research Conference, Durham, N.C.

Sgroi, S.(Ed.) (1982). *Handbook of clinical intervention in child sexual abuse.* Chicago, Il: University of Illinois Press.

Sgroi, S. (Ed.) (1988). *Vulnerable populations: Evaluation and treatment of sexually abused children and adult survivors.* Lexington, MA: Lexington Books.

Shelton, W. (1963). A study of incest. *International Journal of Offender Therapy and Comparative Criminology, 15,* 139-153.

Stern, D. (1985). *The Interpersonal world of the human infant.* NY: Basic Books, Inc.

Sturkie, K. (1983). Structured group treatment for sexually abused children. *Social Work, 28,* 299-308.

Swanson, L. & Biaffio, M.K. (1985). Therapeutic perspectives on father-daughter incest. *American Journal of Psychiatry, 142,* 667-674.

Tubesing, D. (1979). *Stress Skills Training.* Duluth, MN: Whole Person Associates, Inc.

Trepper, T.S. (1989). Intrafamily child sexual abuse. In C.R. Figley (Ed.), *Treating stress in families,* New York: Brunner/Mazel, Inc.

Tufts New England Medical Center, Division of Child Psychiatry (1984). Sexually exploited children: Service and research project. Final report for the Office of Juvenile Justice and Delinquency Prevention. Washington, D.C.: U.S. Department of Justice.

Wheeler, B.L. (1980). The use of paraverbal therapy in treating an abused child. *The Arts in Psychotherapy,* 14, 69-76.

Van der Kolk, B. (1988). The trauma spectrum: The interaction of biological and social events in the genesis of traumatic response. *Journal of Traumatic Stress, 1*(3), 273-290.

When Staff Members Sexually Abuse Children in Residential Care

Robert B. Bloom, PhD

PRECIS

When an agency staff member is accused of sexually abusing a client, the administration is faced with the Solomonic task of balancing the necessity of protecting the child, supporting the staff, and maintaining the integrity and reputation of the agency. This article presents practical suggestions for managing the agency through such a crisis.

It may come as a surprise to the reader that sexual abuse of children in residential care is no longer an issue of any great concern. "Currently the problem of abuse in out-of-home care is not a primary focus, as concern has shifted to other protective service issues" (Nunno and Motz 1988). Matsushima (1990) asserts, "Given the highly visible social environment of the residential treatment center it would seem almost impossible to commit or

This article is based on a paper presented at the annual meeting of the American Association of Children's Residential Centers in St. Petersburg, FL, November, 1990, and is reprinted with permission from Child Welfare, Volume 71(2), March/April 1992, pp. 131-145.

Dr. Bloom may be written at the Jewish Children's Bureau of Chicago, One South Franklin Street, Chicago, IL 60606.

[Haworth co-indexing entry note]: "When Staff Members Sexually Abuse Children in Residential Care." Bloom, Robert B. Co-published simultaneously in *Residential Treatment for Children & Youth* (The Haworth Press, Inc.) Vol. 11, No. 2, 1993, pp. 89-106; and: *The Management of Sexuality in Residential Treatment* (ed: Gordon Northrup) The Haworth Press, Inc., 1993, pp. 89-106.

conceal abusive acts." He goes on to state, "In residential treatment centers for disturbed children, however, outright abuse is not common."

The literature would seem to support Matsushima's claim. The author reviewed the following journals from 1980 to date: *Social Services Index, CHILD WELFARE, Administration in Social Work, Child Abuse and Neglect,* and *Child and Youth Services Review.* One special issue of *Child and Youth Services Review* and eight other articles were the totality of papers on institutional child abuse. Most were conceptual in nature. There were three articles on demography, only one of which concerned itself with institutional abuse in the United States. Only two articles addressed sexual abuse, neither involving residential treatment. There were no articles whatsoever in the administrative literature. Yet the National Center on Child Abuse and Neglect (1978) alleges that "Despite the best intentions of program managers, all too often children are victims of maltreatment in the very institutions which are operated to care for and serve their needs."

In their landmark study, Rindfleisch and Rabb (1984) project that reportable abuse complaints in residential treatment centers may occur at twice the rate at which they occur within families; they indicate that fewer than one in five complainable situations in out-of-home placements is likely to be reported to child protective service agencies.

In his personal experience since 1981, the author knows of nine staff members of four agencies in two different states who sexually abused 12 children in residential treatment. In addition, two "seduction sequences" were uncovered and stopped; and one new staff member was discovered to have been indicted for abusing a handicapped child at another agency. Twelve of 12 allegations were true! It is highly unlikely that the author's experience is unique. The vacuum in the literature may have a much more insidious cause.

Since a specific incident of abuse by an individual worker in an institutional setting is often the result of many circumstances within the institution, accusations of child abuse against an individual are commonly viewed as attacks on the entire institution. The resistance to such reports, therefore, tends to be strong, and the institutions which would welcome them tend to be those that are not likely to have high rates of abuse. Institutions' responses to such external attack may include reactions similar to those manifested in families identified or accused of abuse: denial, cover-up action, or defensive behavior. The motivations for "avoiding" the problems are also similar. The accused will fear punishment or reprisal, want to protect reputations and careers, try to cover the deed to serve the long-term needs of the social unit, and be unwilling to acknowledge the presence of internal factors that lead to child abuse. Whatever the powerful forces that evoke abusive behavior, professional training and understanding do not assure the taking of prompt, positive, and appropriate action. (Durkin 1982)

When a residential staff member is accused of sexually abusing a child, the agency has three concurrent responsibilities. The first and paramount concern is protecting the child-victim and other children. Next, the agency must offer support to the alleged perpetrator and all other staff members. Last in importance, but critical, the agency must take steps to maintain the reputation and integrity of the agency. This article offers practical suggestions on how to manage all three responsibilities.

PROTECTING THE CHILD

The overriding concern must be for the safety, protection, and well-being of the child. Steps must be taken to support the child emotionally and to protect the child from possible attempts at retribution by staff members or peers. Vulnerable children likely to be significantly affected should be identified and supported throughout the abuse-related crisis.

Believe It Can Happen

The single greatest impediment to adequately protecting residential clients from sexual abuse is the attitude that "it can't happen here." It is a common belief that only "bad" agencies, only obviously "sick" people, are involved in residential abuse. The reality is that even those agencies with exceptional risk management policies and procedures are not free from the possibility of employing a high-risk person.

There is some degree of randomness built into the risk. The pressure to employ staff, especially child care staff, can often be intense, leading to procedural shortcuts in hiring. State investigatory systems frequently are overloaded and allow bypass procedures that increase risk. Often there are long time lags between reports–even indictments–and the actual logging of information into the abuse registries. All too frequently some organizations fire abusers and fail to make reports to child protective services; and the current personnel practice of validating[1] employment can make employment reference-checking worthless.

Many sex abusers, by deceit and creative manipulation of others, are able to avoid detection. In one case a nighttime child care worker did not list his previous employment at a state child facility. His personal and other employment references checked out. At his trial it was discovered that he had been discharged from a state agency for abuse of clients. His references turned out to be relatives with different last names. Following a newspaper article about the trial, another state child care facility called to inquire if the person they recently had employed was the person named in the newspaper article! He was, of course.

Take Allegations Seriously

It has been the author's uniform experience that allegations of sexual abuse of residents by staff members are true. Whatever the initial impressions of the allegation may be, the clinically and ethically appropriate response is to listen to the child carefully, courteously, and nondefensively. The incident should be explored openly, candidly, and in an empathic and supportive manner. The interviewer should try to view the incident exactly as the child experienced it by asking open-ended questions about it. The interview should be task-focused and information-gathering. *The child must be helped to help the interviewer see the abusive event from his or her point of view.* Supporting information should be solicited, such as where the event occurred; when; what else was happening at the time; who else might have been in the area. In one situation the child gave so detailed a description of the staff member's apartment that the investigating administrator was able to draw a sketch of the living room. A photograph of the living room was obtained later and corresponded exactly with the drawing.

Suspend the Employee with Pay During the Initial Investigation

The first duty is to protect the child. Removing the potential source of harm–suspending the alleged abuser–clearly demonstrates the agency's commitment to protecting the child. For other types of abuse the author recommends a case-by-case determination of the appropriateness of suspension. Sexual abuse allegations, however, have an insidious impact on the milieu. Many children have their own abuse experiences reawakened. The staff member will not be able to perform his or her job responsibilities. The campus will become so focused on the abuse issue that the program will suffer. Suspending the alleged perpetrator helps to reduce the disruptiveness and anxiety triggered by the allegation as well as protecting the child. In addition, the suspension protects the staff member from allegations of tampering with the evidence or coercing the child.

Reach Out to the Child's Family

The family should be informed of the child's allegations and what is being done about them. The family should be given a description of how their child is being protected, how their child is being helped to work through this crisis, and what services are being provided to their child. The family must be helped to support their child, even if they disbelieve the allegations.[2] The likely series of steps involving child protective services, rape crisis teams, law enforcement, and the courts should be carefully explained to the family. Reaching out to families is not only clinically appropriate and ethically right, it may also reduce the likelihood of a lawsuit.

Act to Cut Off Retribution by Staff Members or Peers

A child alleging sexual abuse by a staff member is frequently scapegoated by peers and staff members. Typically the alleged abuser is well liked by the children, who become angry at and frequently harass the child making the allegations. Staff members may try to dissuade the child from holding to his or her allegations. They may distance themselves emotionally from the child. They may have great difficulty believing the allegations. With adolescents, staff members are likely to blame the victim for seducing the staff member. They will minimize the abusive staff member's illegal behavior if the child has been promiscuous. Without clear and direct intervention the child will most likely be made to feel more guilty, more responsible, and more unable to control his or her life.

A series of well-planned meetings should be held with various groups of the treatment community.

> The executive staff member who suspended the employee should meet with all residential staff members to inform them of what has happened, what steps are being taken, and what steps need to be taken with the victim, other children, and the alleged perpetrator. Everyone needs to be reminded of the primary responsibility to protect the child.

> The alleged victim's treatment team meets with the living-unit peers to allow them to express their feelings, ask questions, and so forth. The team works both on assuring the children that they are safe and in eliciting support for the child making the allegation. The key executive staff member should be available to the children if they want to meet with him or her.

> If the suspended staff person works in a unit other than the one in which the alleged victim lives, the executive who suspended the staff person should meet with the treatment team and children of that unit. A full description and explanation of what has transpired and will transpire should be given to them.

> All units should hold simultaneous house meetings to allow the children to express their feelings, ask questions, be reas-

sured of their own safety, and develop empathy and support for the child victim.

Flood the Child with Support

A multiservice plan should be developed that both symbolically and clinically supports the child through the abuse investigation process and aftermath. If available, an outside rape crisis team should be brought in. The child should see a sexual abuse treatment specialist. Therapy time with the current therapist should be increased as needed. All the significant adults in the life of the child should be available as needed.

To help the child manage the flood of conflicting feelings she or he is experiencing, the agency must unambiguously side with the child until such time as it is proven clearly that the abuse did not occur. Support will be clearly demonstrated to the child by the agency's full cooperation with investigatory and prosecutory agents. The child should be helped to tell his or her story to parents, child protective service workers, police, and prosecuting attorneys.

Because so many residential clients themselves have been sexually abused, many children will experience the same panoply of frightening feelings as the victim. Treatment teams should review all children in their care in order to identify the vulnerable children. Vulnerable children should be given whatever additional treatment or supportive time they need from the staff.

SUPPORTING THE STAFF

When a staff member is accused of sexually abusing a resident child, feelings of anger, fear, anxiety, distrust, and guilt can radiate across an agency like the aftershocks of a major earthquake. Where trust has been established, relationships are shaken; where there is no trust, relationships are fractured. Old issues resurface. Racial tension, union-management conflicts, and employee-supervisor problems can create a deleterious undercurrent that interferes with the agency's ability to treat the children in its care. While clearly affirming its primary duty to the children, the agency must safeguard the rights and dignity of the alleged abuser. And it publicly must communicate this intention to the staff.

Allow the Alleged Abuser to Tell His or Her Story in the Same Manner and by Using the Same Interviewing Techniques Used with the Child

Everyone has a right to be heard in an empathic, fair, and impartial manner. Everyone should be heard and each one's story given due consideration. Even though the alleged abuser will be suspended, the incident must be explored with him or her in a direct, open, candid, and nonthreatening manner. The purpose is not to conduct a criminal investigation; rather, enough information must be gathered to allow the agency to make the best treatment and management decisions for the child, the alleged abuser, and the agency.

Treat the Abuser with Respect and Dignity

Neither the child nor the agency is well-served by treating the alleged abuser, even when guilty, in a demeaning and psychologically abusive manner. Handling of the alleged perpetrator should be done with the expectation that everything said or done to the staff member will become public knowledge. The administrator's sense of fair play, its basic human decency, will be judged by the staff according to the way the alleged abuser is treated.

Explain the Suspension as Meeting the Agency's Primary Duty to Assure the Safety of the Child

The alleged abuser and the other staff members are certain to view the suspension as a conviction without a trial. They must constantly be reminded of their primary duty to protect and advocate for children. The staff should be told that should the allegations prove to be untrue the agency will do all it can to undo the harm done to the alleged abuser.

Maintain the Alleged Abuser's Wage and Benefit Status Until the Time That the Abuser May Have to be Discharged

No one is ever made psychologically whole following an allegation that he or she sexually abused a child. Of necessity, the process must be skewed toward protecting the child. The agency should, however, protect the employee's financial status until convinced the abuse occurred. Treating the alleged abuser fairly signals to all the staff members what they can expect from the agency should they find themselves in difficult situations.

Explain the Alleged Abuser's Due Process Rights and Indicate a Willingness to Help the Person to Use Them

The agency and union grievance procedures should be carefully explained to the alleged abuser. The employee should be informed that irrespective of the grievance procedures he or she might want to consult an attorney, and also should be asked if he or she needs help to initiate grievance procedures or to locate an attorney. The help should be provided if it is requested.

Convene an All-Residential Meeting of Child Care Workers, Therapists, Teachers, Administrators, Supervisors, and the Support Staff

The agency must appear to be in full charge of the process. It must be clear that the agency, not child protective services, is making all of the personnel decisions. The agency must be viewed as fair, ethical, and caring for all members of its residential community. The best way to calm the emotional undercurrent is to communicate to the staff clearly and unambiguously what has been done, and what will be done in response to the abuse allegations. An all-staff meeting is an effective way to help settle the campus. In the meeting, the staff should be told what allegations have been made, who made them, and about who they were made.[3]

> As much information as possible should be given. Staff members should be told what legal and other constraints restrict the agency's ability to give them a fuller account.

The staff should be reminded of the agency's duty to protect and advocate for children.

How the alleged abuser's due process rights will be protected and enabled should be described. A description should be given of how the agency will protect the alleged abuser's financial status, and an explanation should be given of what the agency will do if the allegations turn out to be false.

Lots of time must be allowed for staff members to vent their feelings, to ask questions, or to challenge the administrator's actions.

Staff members' feelings of anger, frustration, and vulnerability must be identified, validated, and supported.

The administration must maintain an open door policy. Key administrators should be available to each and every staff person who wants to discuss the issues privately.

Prepare the Staff to Deal with the Anticipated Behavior and Feelings of the Children

A certain amount of staff members' anxiety will be related to their concern about how the children now will respond to them. Staff members will also be concerned about how to respond appropriately to their children's heightened emotional needs for support and nurturance. Inservice training should be provided promptly on how to minimize peer retribution against the victim, handle children's anger toward the staff, and respond to the children's stirred-up feelings about their own abuse experiences.

Keep the Staff Fully Informed as Events Happen, But Keep the Focus on Supporting Children and Getting on with the Treatment Program

Everyone will want to know what is happening–the status of the alleged perpetrator and the child. Staff members will want to share impressions of how their children are responding to the crisis. Although the staff must be kept informed, abusive incidents can drain time, energy, and resources from the operation of the regular program. It is not uncommon for basic program elements to be ignored. It develops somehow that there is no time to take children shopping for clothing, snacks, or personal items. Recreational activity programming is often truncated. The heightened emotional climate may lead the staff to believe the community access must be curtailed, that everyone should remain on the campus until "things have settled down." In a very short time the carefully structured and integrated 24-hour program becomes fragmented. The milieu then not only can lose its treatment impact, it can become a countertherapeutic agent leading to much acting out by the children, with concomitant reactive restrictive behavior by the staff. Despite the importance of providing the staff with ongoing information about the abusive situation, the administrators and supervisors must ensure the normal operation of the basic 24-hour treatment program.

MAINTAINING THE ORGANIZATION

Although the primary duties are first to protect the children, and second to support the staff, the best management of those responsibilities will also prove to be critical in restoring the equilibrium of the agency, as well as reducing the likelihood of litigation. Responding directly and unambiguously in the best interests of the alleged child victim is vital to maintaining the agency's treatment integrity and its reputation as a good place for the care of troubled children. How an agency reacts will be given much greater emphasis by protective services, clients, and referral sources than the occurrence of the abusive event. Handling the alleged abuser in a fair and humane way will help to maintain the reputation of the agency as a good place in which to work. A series of other administrative decisions must be made.

Fight the Compulsion to Deny, Cover Up, and Defend

While there is widespread agreement among administrators of children's facilities that program monitoring, professional rapport with the residents, and an "open door" policy are sufficient to assure the safety and security of residents, reporting of maltreatment has been negligible. (Rindfleisch 1988)

Not only are there very strong emotional forces to act defensively, there are real concerns about the reputation, future, and fiscal liabilities of the agency. The best defense may be a good offense. Forthright, unambiguous management of the abuse-related circumstances, paired with clear and direct communication of the agency's response to the situation, will help to counteract the natural tendencies to be secretive and defensive.

Inform the "Shareholders"

There are many interested parties, "shareholders," of a child-caring agency–the board of directors, major referral sources, clients, staff members, and the community at large. All are entitled to candid and unambiguous communication from the agency administration.

Executive staff. Whether directly involved in the residential program or not, all key staff members must be informed. They no doubt are part of extensive community and professional networks. They must be able to respond accurately to inquiries about what the agency is doing in response to the allegation.

Executive committee of the board of directors. It should be obvious that the key lay leadership must be fully informed. If the abusive event is at all likely to become known in the community, the whole board should be informed. By sharing everything with the lay leadership the executive director shares the burden, engenders support and creative problem-solving assistance, and solidifies, rather than weakens, his or her relationship with the board of directors.

Major referral sources. Referral sources are very likely to learn about the abuse allegation. Rather than allow them to get a sure-to-be-distorted view, the agency should provide its major referral sources with full details on how the agency is handling the situation. Instead of being put in the position of panicky overseers, their "shareholders" status should be enhanced by soliciting their input and assistance. At one agency, the failure to work cooperatively with the local child services agency was one critical variable in the referring agency's decision to precipitously remove all its clients.

Union. Forthright and timely communication with the union will minimize the stress on labor-management relationships. The union should be informed whenever a bargaining unit member is accused of sexual abuse of a resident. In all likelihood the agency's labor contract requires that the union be informed whenever severe disciplinary action is to be taken against a union member. In this instance, because of the emergency nature of this situation, the union member may have to be suspended without following the usual disciplinary due process requirements of the contract. Since the union is often a collective of child welfare professionals, they will, if allowed, be truly concerned about the safety and well-being of children in care and support agency efforts in managing the crisis activities.

Have One Clearly Visible, Accessible, Senior Manager in Charge of Managing the Process

To respond adequately to the multitude of constituencies; to meet the needs of the children, the staff, and the program; and to manage the pressures generated by the abusive incident will require an inordinate amount of administrative time. To keep the communication processes open, coordinate and oversee the series of activities, and demonstrate that the agency is effectively managing the process, one senior administrator should be designated as the person in charge. All information and communication should be channeled to this person. The designated coordinator will need regular access to, and support from, the executive director and the cabinet or management committee of the agency. For a large multiservice agency, the director of residential treatment is the logical choice. For a small or solely residential service agency, the executive director is a sensible choice. When the crisis coordinator is not the executive director, communication networks with the board of directors will need to be established.

Be Prepared for Legal Action

Initiate liability-reducing strategies before anyone threatens or takes legal action against the agency. Planning should anticipate legal action from the abused child, the suspected staff member, and the union. If some angry persons contact particular organizations, the agency may be faced with reviews by a variety of licensing and oversight bodies.[4] The old saying, "If it isn't written down it didn't happen," applies in any type of liability risk-management situation. Therefore, document what has been done to protect the child and to support the rights of the alleged abuser. Communication activities with the "shareholders" should also be documented.

The agency's attorney must be informed. Because he or she is likely to advise the administration to say nothing to anyone about the alleged abuse, the agency may well find itself in a conflict between good clinical practice, good personnel management, and even good risk management, on the one hand, and its attorney's recommendations, on the other. The author's suggestion is to inform the agency's attorney of its crisis management plan and ask that a legal strategy be developed that recognizes the need to run the agency in a way that provides for the protection of the children, the support of the staff, and the maintenance of the agency's integrity and reputation.

The agency's insurance carrier must be informed. Frightening insurance companies is not the best way to curtail premiums, but the agency's carriers must be promptly informed. Insurance companies have been known to refuse to pay in liability situations where they believe that communication with them was not timely. The risk of the agency actually losing its insurance umbrella may not be great; should that happen, however, the impact will be catastrophic.

Be Prepared for a Trial in the Media

The abuse event, especially if sensational enough in their view, will be covered by the media. Trials, being public, increase the likelihood of media coverage. Should the media become involved, the coordinating administrator should be made available to them. The media should be provided with the same information as everyone else about the steps being taken both to protect the children and to prevent recurrences of abusive incidents. The agency should want its story to be given to the media. Basic protective instinct, professional beliefs about confidentiality, and the agency's attorney all will urge silence, but if the agency remains silent it will be convicted in the media. Residential sexual abuse can happen anywhere. The media generally know this, but if they do not, the agency should try to teach them. In a manner similar to the way referral sources will evaluate the agency, the media and public will judge the agency by how it handles the situation.

> The agency must always appear to be open, helpful, and cooperative. It should never lie. As Mark Twain said, "Always tell the truth. It will surprise some and gratify the rest."

> The agency must never say, "No comment." No comment will be taken as a confession that the agency is the worst kind of snake pit for children. Only straightforward communication has any chance of reducing the distortion rampant in media coverage.

> Admit that there has been an allegation. If there has been a system glitch, such as the alleged abuser being hired without all of the required checks, or based on wrong information, it should be admitted. To such an admission should be added a description of the steps being taken to correct the problem and to avoid similar problems in the future. Everyone makes mistakes. The public will respect frankness, especially when presented with clear action plans to help the child and prevent recurrences.

A few comments about confidentiality:

> It is no breach of confidentiality to discuss matters that are already public.

> It is no breach of confidentiality to describe procedures.

If there is a criminal trial, the record and proceedings are open to the public. The records of civil proceedings are also open to the public.

Although breach of confidentiality by the alleged victim may open issues for comment, specific client-related facts should not be discussed. Nevertheless, the opening can be used by the agency to demonstrate that its policies, procedures, and practices are sensible and represent competent treatment of children in residential care. Suppose, for example, the client tells the media that a "child care worker used to drive me in his car when I went home on visits, and we had sex in the car. The supervisor never knew when he left or how long he was gone or what he was doing." In its response the agency can comment on its policy regarding staff members driving children, why it needs to be done, how it is supervised and documented, and how staff members have driven thousands of miles without incident to take children home, to hospitals, to doctors, to the many other places to which children must be taken.

Seek Institutional Factors That Could Enable the Behavior to Take Place

Prevention begins with a clear policy statement that the agency's mission is protecting and caring for children, and that any sexual activity between staff members and clients of any age is forbidden and will lead to dismissal and criminal prosecution. The agency must attack misguided loyalty on the part of workers by making it clear that it will not tolerate passive acceptance or an unwillingness of staff members to intervene when an employee behaves inappropriately with clients.

Although prevention is not the focus of this paper, it is importance to note that the abusive situation should serve as a signal to initiate a risk management analysis of the agency. This typically is not done. "Response occurs to the abuse incident, but little attention is given to the institution beyond the investigation and substantiation of the incident" (Kelleher 1987).

A competent risk management analysis should review hiring practices, orientation, training, supervision, and articulated philosophy. The communication network should also be reviewed. The communication network in a residential treatment center is a principal safeguard against abuse of residents. The agency should make certain that its network is an open system in which information flows freely. Everyone must understand his or her duty to report any and all abusive incidents.

CONCLUSION

Sexual abuse of children in residential care constitutes a horrible breach of trust. The effects can be devastating for children, staff members, and agencies. Managing the agency during such apocalyptic times feels very much like a lose-lose situation. Time, effort, money, and energy are consumed at enormous rates.

The silver lining is hard to find in these clouds. This article suggests that in responding to abusive incidents, agencies can reaffirm basic human values of caring and justice in a manner that demonstrates integrity and competence as a child-caring agency.

NOTES

1. Validation policy dictates that in response to a reference check a previous employer give only the dates, salary, and job description for a former employee.

2. If, as is likely, the child has been a victim of intrafamilial sex abuse, the associated pain and anxiety will return. Intensive treatment services must be made available to reestablish the family's homeostasis to at least the level of functioning before the allegations. The crisis may provide an opportunity to revitalize stalled treatment.

3. The author found the staff very appreciative of this approach. At negotiation time, however, the union used it to demonstrate that the alleged abusers were convicted without a fair hearing. Fortunately, the staff knew better.

4. This kind of action typically is initiated by disgruntled staff members. Open communication and fair practice with the staff militates against such a development.

REFERENCES

Durkin, R. "No One Will Thank You: First Thoughts on Reporting Institutional Abuse." Child and Youth Services Review IV, 1, 2 (1982): 109-113.

Kelleher, M. E. "Investigating Institutional Abuse: A Post-Substantiation Model." CHILD WELFARE LXVI, 4 (July-August 1987): 343-351.

Matsushima, J. "Interviewing for Alleged Abuse in the Residential Treatment Center." CHILD WELFARE LXIX, 4 (July-August 1990): 321-331.

National Center on Child Abuse and Neglect. Child Abuse and Neglect in Residential Institutions: Selected Readings on Prevention, Investigation, and Correction. Washington DC: National Center on Child Abuse and Neglect, 1978.

Nunno, M. A., and Motz, J. K. "The Development of an Effective Response to the Abuse of Children in Out-of-Home Care." Child Abuse and Neglect 12 (1988): 521-528.

Rindfleisch, N. Political Obstacles to Reporting in Residential Care Settings. In Professional Responsibilities in Protecting Children, edited by A. Manye and S. Wells. New York: Praeger, 1988.

Rindfleisch, N., and Rabb, J. "How Much of a Problem is Residential Mistreatment in Child Welfare Institutions?" Child Abuse and Neglect 8 (1984): 33-40.

Erotic Countertransference Issues in a Residential Treatment Center

Danilo E. Ponce, MD

SUMMARY. Treating youngsters who are moderately to severely psychiatrically disordered in institutional settings often arouses in staff intense sexual feelings. This paper focuses on the nature of these feelings and how these may be dealt with clinically and administratively. "Erotic" rather than "sexual" is the preferred term used in the paper to indicate the view that although some of these reactions are, in the final analysis, indeed sexual in nature, the way they are manifested usually assumes many deceptive forms. That is to say, some of the reactions may be overtly sexual, but others take the form of innocent looking affiliative actions such as "too much hugging," "too much spoiling," or to use a currently favored term—"too much bonding."

To borrow a graphic metaphor that has been used in describing the dynamics of alcoholism in a family (Simpkinson, 1990), the issue of erotic countertransference reactions (hereafter referred to as ECR's) by staff in a residential treatment center (hereafter referred to as RTC) is like that of "an elephant parked in the family living room": it is obvious enough so you can't miss it, it is conspicuous enough so you can't avoid it, its influence is compelling enough so that you can't dismiss it—and yet everybody somehow manages to

The author may be written at University of Hawaii, John A. Burns Medical School, Department of Psychiatry, Honolulu, HI.

[Haworth co-indexing entry note]: "Erotic Countertransference Issues in a Residential Treatment Center." Ponce, Danilo E. Co-published simultaneously in *Residential Treatment for Children & Youth* (The Haworth Press, Inc.) Vol. 11, No. 2, 1993, pp. 107-123 and: *The Management of Sexuality in Residential Treatment* (ed: Gordon Northrup) The Haworth Press, Inc., 1993, pp. 107-123. Multiple copies of this article/chapter may be purchased from The Haworth Document Delivery Center [1-800-3-HAWORTH; 9:00 a.m. - 5:00 p.m. (EST)].

tiptoe gingerly around it, ignore it, or pretend that it does not exist. Times are rapidly changing, however, so that like it or not RTCs (or for that matter, any institutions that are involved in caring for or treating youngsters for an extended period of time) can no longer afford to play hide and seek with this elephant in the living room.

Patients, parents, and at times other staff members are increasingly taking the initiative in reporting incidents of alleged sexual misconduct on the part of staff towards the youngsters, spurred on, no doubt, by community outrage, and the vigorous zeal on the part of prosecutors to pursue these charges (Time, 1990; U.S. News and World Report, 1990). Literature on the subject is just now beginning to trickle in (see for example Schneider, 1985; Realmuto, 1986), and academic interest in a subject is usually a good index of mounting anxiety over it, or at least, an uneasy portent of things to come. There is some urgency, therefore, to focus our collective attention on ECR issues. Otherwise, we could conceivably find ourselves in a similar gridlock as now exists in so-called "physical abuse" of patients by staff, where there is considerable debate and acrimony about when legitimate "therapeutic physical containment" ends, and "physical abuse" of the patient begins.

"Erotic," as used in the paper will mean a wide range of feelings, reactions, attitudes, and behaviors that includes the blatantly sexual (e.g., fondling of breasts or genitalia, french kissing, frotteurism, and sexual intercourse), to the subtly sexual that deceptively masquerades as affiliative acts of care and compassion (e.g., "spoiling," "too much hugging/kissing," and pseudointimacy). These reactions could be construed as going above and beyond the expectable and conventional show of therapeutic empathy and affection toward the youngsters, but are never quite gross enough as to be labelled "sexual."

"Countertransference" is a harder concept to pin down since opinions vary as to what it is (Cohen, 1952). Freud (1910) initially introduced the term to describe the analyst's "transference" reactions toward the *analysand*; "transference" in turn being the *projection* of feelings and attitudes from figures in the analysand's past to the analyst. For some inexplicable reason, Freud treated countertransference phenomena merely as an *impediment* in *analysis*, and did not have much to say about it—certainly, not as much as he had to say about transference phenomena (Sandler et al., 1970). As a result of this "neglect," there is now a lack of consensus as to what would be a proper understanding and use of the term in clinical practice. Be that as it may, there are three general ways in which the term is currently being used professionally (Perkins et al., 1984):

1. *Classical*–feelings and attitudes of analysts that are for the most part unconscious, representing reactions from past figures, and projected into the analysand;
2. *Totalistic*–all feelings and attitudes of *care-giving staff* towards their patients, clients, students, or wards; and
3. *Complementary*–a natural, role responsive, necessary counterpart to the transference of the patient.

At the risk of sounding as though I am resurrecting antiquated issues that are no longer clinically relevant, (Marcus, 1980), it needs to be emphasized that transference/countertransference concepts originally referred *only* to phenomena observed in the *analytical situation*, and were not intended to be used willy-willy in any other context (e.g., "therapy," institutionalized "care-giving"). Although it is beyond the scope of this paper to go into the implications of the latter in detail, it does make a significant difference whether we are dealing with erotic countertransference as it occurs in "analysis," "therapy," or being a "staff" in a treatment center. I will deal with these significant differences later on when I discuss the clinical implications. For now, erotic countertransference reactions as presented in the paper shall refer primarily to line staff in care-giving and treatment centers for children and youth, utilizing the meanings described earlier. It is also important to note that countertransference reactions apply equally well to impulses to *do* erotic acts with the youngsters (e.g., sexual intercourse), as well as to strong impulses to *avoid doing* acts that may have erotic connotations (e.g., absolutely refusing to do bedchecks at night).

Initially, I will present a model of talking about ECR–basically an adaption of Marshall's (1979) typology of countertransference with children and adolescents. Where appropriate, I will provide clinical vignettes to illustrate a type or a point being made. Following discussion of the various types, I will then explore the implications of ECR in overall program operations, and conclude with some recommendations on how to address the issue in a clinical as well as an administrative context.

EROTIC COUNTERTRANSFERENCE REACTIONS IN A RTC

Marshall's (1979) typology of countertransference phenomena is a succinct, yet quite lucid and practical way of discussing ECRs in a RTC setting. Marshall's schema originally referred to nonspecific countertransference reactions with children and adolescents, within the context of the "therapist-patient" dyad. Setting aside these differences for the time being, ECRs in a RTC may be seen as occurring in a two by two grid, which establishes two broad groupings:

	Unconscious	Conscious
Staff-Induced ECRs	Type	Type II
Patient-Induced ECRs	Type III	Type IV

Type I: Staff-Induced ECRs–Unconscious

Marshall considers this form the most pernicious and potentially the most problematic to deal with, since it is unconscious and originates from the staff. Perkins (Perkins et al., 1984) cites two common forms:

A. Benign exploitation–This is usually manifested as a compelling need to help, be needed, or to be indispensable to the youngster. Youngsters are psychologically set up to go along with the staff's needs "or else . . . " This is the so-called "missionary position" of pseudointimacy, as well as erotic rescue fantasies. The staff member exhibits many erotic behaviors or equivalents towards the youngsters (e.g., hugging, kissing, stroking, massaging). The implicit but unmistakable message is "Let me take care of your sexual needs."

Clinical vignette: Female staff member in her early forties felt that the female adolescent patients were mainly victims of male physical and sexual exploitation, and that the male staff members merely perpetuated this pattern in the center. She took it upon herself to "correct" this situation by being overly physically demonstrative with the patients. Although some staff began expressing questions about possible "lesbian" themes in her behaviors, the issue was never fully discussed in the open, until she was finally asked to resign for reasons other than concerns around sexual issues.

Clinical vignette: Male staff member in his mid twenties became convinced that what the female patient in her late teens needs was the "loving care of a mature man." He saw himself as providing the "loving care," resigned his position to pursue his mission to save the patient, and convinced the patient (who was by now 18 yrs. old) to live with him upon discharge.

B. Projective exploitation—Projection of staff's unconscious erotic needs onto the patient. The underlying message is "Because I did not get my erotic needs satisfied when I was growing up, I know what it must be like, with you. Hence, I will insure that you do not experience what I experienced by satisfying your erotic needs." This type has the most potential for a catastrophic and tragic outcome, since it lays the foundation for justifying overt sexual behaviors towards the patients (i.e., "acting out") under the altruistic rationale of being "therapeutic" with them.

Clinical vignette: Male staff member in his fifties made a practice of talking to female adolescent patients about details of male/female sexual arousal behaviors, ostensibly to "sexually educate them." His supervisor began to get complaints from the patients, and the possibility that he was getting "titillated by titillating" brought out in supervision. The staff member became indignant and resigned shortly thereafter.

Clinical vignette: Female staff member in her mid twenties would reportedly get "spiritual messages" that would instruct her to help latency-age male patients "become men" by masturbating or performing oral sex on them.

Type II: Staff-Induced ECRs–Conscious

This includes all Type I reactions, except that the staff member "knows" or is aware at some level of the erotic feelings, possible origin of the feelings, and possible outcomes if the feelings are given free reign and "acted out." And yet, despite this awareness, staff seems powerless to do something about the feelings. Perkins (1984) warns that because there is a modicum of awareness of what is going on, there is the danger of dismissing these reactions in a cavalier manner, chalking it up to "individual stylistic differences." It is as if being aware and admitting the feelings publicly would somehow justify or mitigate their being acted out. Thus, one hears staff quite often saying "I can't help it . . . I'm a naturally demonstrative person, and I know some kids and maybe some staff might misinterpret my actions, but that's the way I am." This is also where so-called "cultural differences" regarding "what is merely exotic vs. what is really erotic" gets played out, and become potential sources of problematic interstaff conflicts (e.g., "Where I come from, we feel that children need to be hugged and touched a lot. I'm awfully sorry that you come from a very uptight culture, but I'm not going to stop, just because you object to my hugging and touching the kids.")

This type therefore presents a most perplexing administrative dilemma. It lends itself well to conceptual, moral, or legal double-binds because staff is aware, at least on the surface, of the actual or potential erotic possibilities in an incident or a situation, while at the same time the administrator tries to avoid confronting it *without appearing to do so*. This feat of mental legerdemain is accomplished with seemingly logical "yes, ... " For example, should staff do "bed-checks" to insure that no sexual activities are going on amongst the residents, or should the residents have the "right to privacy"? Should staff intervene when "John and Lisa are getting it on," or should staff look the other way and simply dismiss it as "normal developmental heterosexual behavior"? If so, should homosexual behaviors also be ignored since they are no longer automatically considered as "pathological"? Should talking about pubertal issues (e.g., secondary sexual characteristics, ejaculations, menses, etc.) be commonplace in treatment considerations, or is the "private" and "personal" information best left to "doctors" and "therapists"? What about dress codes? Since contemporary community standards are quite liberal, shouldn't the institution reflect the community standards?

On the surface, the dilemmas engendered by Type II ECRs appear to be valid, and potentially insoluble. Closer inspection, however, reveals that the dilemmas are subtle distractions from the real task at hand, which is what to do about the *erotic countertransference reactions*. The institution should be careful not to get enmeshed in seemingly legitimate arguments about the "pros" and "cons" of dealing with Type II ECRs and instead, recognize that these could be massive avoidance mechanisms working to avoid confronting the issue head-on.

Type III: Patient-Induced ECRs–Unconscious

As in Type I, the youngster is quite capable of benign or projective exploitation of staff which is capable of arousing ECRs in staff. This is classic transference/countertransference situation. In benign exploitation, staff is the recipient of seductive stroking, rubs, massages, etc., under the guise of ". . . you poor thing you . . . you've been working too hard . . . let me rub your neck and make you feel a little better." In projective exploitation Type III, a youngster seeks, for example, to empower staff perceived as "impotent," by offering herself/himself as the vehicle for staff's empowerment and staff responds with ECR. It is important to remember that we are primarily speaking here of *staff's* ECR reactions, which are stemming from the patient's unconscious provocations.

> **Clinical vignette:** Adolescent female patient kept staying up late to chat with a young (early twenties) male night staff member who was relatively new on the job. She would tell him that he was "unlike the rest of the staff" because he was "patient, understanding, and seemed to be quite 'together.'" Eventually, patient started confiding to him her "problems"

with her own sexuality, and implied that only the staff member could "help" her. They started frenchkissing in the staff office, but reportedly, it did not lead to intercourse or ejaculation. Patient eventually let on to other staff what happened. The staff member was quite irate and threatened legal action when he was asked to resign because he felt he was "set up" by the patient.

Type IV: Patient-Induced ECRs–Conscious

This type is the paradigm of the optimal therapeutic use of ECRs whereby:

A. Staff is experiencing erotic reactions;
B. Staff is fully aware and understands that the stimulus is coming from the youngster's habitual and perhaps psychopathological mode of relating; and
C. Staff uses his/her erotic responses for diagnostic and/or therapeutic purposes. This type would correspond to the third meaning of countertransference mentioned earlier–the complementary type of ECRs.

> **Team Psychiatrist:** "I find Clarissa (not her real name) an extremely sexually attractive and provocative young woman. I find myself wondering that if she has this effect on me, how much more so with her stepfather?"

> **Social Worker:** He's got that "lost little boy look," kinda wants me to just hold him in my arms, let him cry his heart out, so I can say to him, "There . . . there it's OK . . . I'll take care of everything." "I think you all (staff) must have had these feelings too, but maybe you weren't quite sure whether it would be okay to have these feelings or not."

CLINICAL IMPLICATIONS

At the outset, I mentioned that it was important to note that the concepts of transference/countertransference were originally intended to apply to phenomena observed between the analyst and the analysand (and in a much less clearer way, to the therapist and the patient) in the analytic situation. As such, there were built-in safeguards, albeit implicit, to insure that both phenomena were not to be ignored, trifled with, or acted out. With staff in caregiving or treatment institutions, these safeguards are virtually nonexistent for the following reasons:

1. *Moderate to Severely Psychiatrically Disordered Adolescent Population*–In analysis, the "patient" (analysand), is usually young, affluent, verbal, intelligent, sophisticated, has a relatively normal family and support system, and is in the analytic situation of his/her own accord. Youngsters in RTCs on the other hand are usually highly disturbed, impulsive, have an abusive/abused history (physical and sexual), with very dysfunctional family and support systems, and are resistant to the RTC placement. With sex and sexuality as their core developmental and psychopathological issues, these youngsters are quite adept, therefore, at eliciting ECRs whether as recipients or inducers.
2. *Immature, Untrained, and Inexperienced Staff*–Analysts and therapists undergo long periods of schooling and training where one of the requirements is extensive self-examination for the express purpose of minimizing unconscious ECRs. There is usually no such training or requirement necessary to be a staff in a RTC.
3. *Analytic/Therapeutic Alliance*–In analysis and therapy, there is the careful cultivation of the "alliance" which provides the matrix within which transference/countertransference reactions are dealt with safely and professionally. There is no such "alliance" between staff and patients, other than the usual and quite generic "agreement" that the staff, being representative of the treating institution, will at least "do no harm (primum non nocere)." In a figurative sense, the difference between the presence of an active therapeutic alliance, and a relatively absent alliance, is like the existence of the "incest taboo" between a biological parent and his/her child, versus the relatively "weak" taboo in a foster parent and a foster child.

4. *Analytic/Therapeutic Commitment*–Staff are less involved in treatment planning, and therefore see their role as peripheral. From a career standpoint, they really see their job as a transitional one. Hence, there is really no strong incentive to do an extensive self-examination to enhance their professional effectiveness. Conversely, their countertransference reactions are generally seldom scrutinized. The reverse is obviously true for analysts and therapists.

5. *Institutional Treatment Philosophies*–Not all RTCs subscribe to the psychosocial framework of treating adolescents. Some are more or less "biological" in orientation relying primarily on psychopharmacology as the main treatment tool. In this context, there is very little need to examine staff reactions, and therefore ECRs are either never mentioned, or if they are acted out, quickly dealt with in a punitive and surreptitious fashion.

Because of these conditions, the possibility of staff acting out their ECRs in RTCs is quite high in my estimation, and is probably already happening, to a certain extent, but not yet fully recognized. By now the theme of the paper should be quite clear–that ECRs by RTC staff are to be expected, that these reactions are probably "catastrophes waiting to happen," and that the prudent position to take is to begin putting into place clinical and administrative safeguards on the well known principle that "an ounce of prevention is worth a pound of cure."

A necessary starting point in addressing this issue is the basic principle that administrative structure and clinical practice must complement and closely interdigitate with each other if the issue is to be addressed successfully. The ease with which ECR issues are dealt with clinically, for instance, will depend on the climate that exists administratively. As an example, if it is an institutional policy that new staff are informed right from the start that ECRs are "to be expected," and that these reactions will be the subject of on-going training, monitoring, and supervision–then an administrative context is created that will be conducive to bringing up and dealing with these reactions in a most "natural" way.

Turning now to specific clinical implications, ECRs could be used diagnostically as data that could indicate the youngster's developmental stage, or the nature of his/her psychopathology. For instance, if staff feels a fairly intense and consistent feeling "to take care of the poor baby, and protect him from the rest of the nasty kids," this could mean that the youngster may be operating predominantly in the "oral" stage of Freudian psychosexual development; on the other hand, a youngster who consistently "teases" staff sexually to get what he/she wants might be exhibiting an adaptive, albeit negative "Initiative" in the Ericksonian developmental scheme.

This is not to imply that *all* erotic reactions by staff are countertransferential in nature, nor do they always indicate in a role-responsive, complementary manner, the youngster's psychopathology or developmental stage. The point is that if enough of a pattern of ECRs from various staff emerges, then certainly this is valuable data that could be used clinically.

It should be evident that these kinds of clinical data are not the usual "objective" data gained through "tests" or "observations," because they are dependent on staff volunteering "sensitive" information about themselves (Beitman, 1983). Realistically, it will take years of concerted effort by senior staff doing role-modeling, and "permission-granting" to foster the kind of clinical atmosphere that will allow staff to use ECRs as valuable clinical tools.

Aside from using ECR for diagnostic purposes, they could also be used clinically as stimulus for special treatment planning, and as a focus for on-going in-service training of staff. It is in this context that Type II issues such as "bedchecks," "dress codes," "how much hugging/kissing is too much," "sexual intercourse among patients," "spoiling," "favoritism," "cross-cultural styles," etc., could be brought out and resolved consciously and professionally.

ADMINISTRATIVE IMPLICATIONS

As with any potentially destructive phenomena that must be paid attention to, and that needs to be handled delicately because of the sensibilities involved, the first administrative step to take is to create what Book (Book et al., 1978) refers to as " . . . the nurturing of an attitude among staff which will minimize the growth of countertransference responses; and to the openness and honesty by which countertransference responses are identified and understood when they do occur." In my experience, there are three basic messages that must be communicated consciously, continuously and consistently over time to staff if this "attitude" is to evolve:

1. ECRs are naturally occurring responses to youngsters' developmental and psychopathological issues.
2. Administrative mechanisms and procedures are available that will assist staff to identify when (not if) they do occur.
3. Administrative support and assistance is available to deal with these reactions in a therapeutic manner.

There is really no need to create a new set of "policies" or "procedures" to communicate these messages effectively, since all one has to do is to take advantage of already existing administrative mechanisms. Examples of these mechanisms are:

1. *In-Service Training*–ECR issues should be part of the orientation training of all new staff, as well as the regular and periodic on-going training curriculum for staff, supervisors, and administrators.
2. *Policies, Procedures, Practices*–There should be (a) clear and explicit policy statements that anticipate ECRs, (b) procedures designed to assist staff with their ECRs, and (c) established practices to handle these reactions in case they are acted out.
3. *Treatment Team and Staff Meetings*–ECR issues should be an on-going agenda in Treatment Team and Staff meetings. This will insure visibility, and continuity. Hopefully, staff will get "desensitized" enough sooner or later and come to accept the issue as part and parcel of day-to-day clinical work.
4. *Staff "Process" Meetings*–Time must be set aside periodically to process ECR issues from an individual as well as a collective basis, in staff meetings. It must be understood that the goal of these process meetings is to get a better clinical understanding *as it relates to diagnosis and treatment planning* of the youngsters. These process meetings should not be allowed to stray into processing of staff "psychopathology." The latter is

best handled in supervision or recommendation for professional assistance.

5. *Supervision*–All supervisors should be expected as a matter of policy to bring up ECR issues as a regular topic in ongoing supervision of their supervisees. Needless to say, this can only happen if there is the proper "attitude" of professionalism mentioned earlier.

6. *Patient Group Meetings*–It is not enough to deal with ECR issues in meetings or mechanisms where only staff are involved. The other, and perhaps more substantial half of the effort, is the involvement of the patients in collectively addressing the issues. Again, ECRs should *not* be treated as a "special" area but presented as merely one among many clinical/administrative areas of concern needing their input and assistance. Naturally-occurring patient group meetings might be the "Health, Sex-Education Meeting," "Therapy Groups," "Cottage-Unit Group Meetings."

7. *Quality Assurance/Risk Management*–These are agency-wide mechanisms where ECR issues should be monitored and dealt with on an on-going basis, as part and parcel of cost-effectiveness and quality control. By making ECR issues quality assurance and risk-management concerns, it reinforces the "attitude" that ECR issues are important factors of consideration in that particular institution.

Raising the agency's consciousness regarding ECR issues by "nurturing an attitude" is merely the first step, albeit the most important step to take administratively. The second step is to extend this attitude of openness regarding ECR issues to the wider network of "consumers"– the parents/significant others, referral sources, third-party payers, etc. Involving this network of consumers before ECRs are acted out has the salutary effect of impressing the consumers: (1) That the agency is in control of the situation by anticipating occurrence of potentially negative behaviors by staff; and (2) that the agency is demonstrating impeccable professionalism by letting them know that mechanisms that identify, monitor, and deal with potential ECRs are in place. Recommended ways of involving consumers are periodic group meetings (e.g., "family nights") and newsletters.

It not only makes good clinical sense to involve consumers, but it also makes for a decided advantage in the unfortunate event of litigation. In these litigious times, the agency must skillfully negotiate between the Scylla of being sued by a disgruntled staff on one hand, and the Charybdis of being sued by patients, irate parents, watchdog agencies, third-party payers, etc., on the other. As an example, if an agency does not have any of the administrative and clinical mechanisms suggested earlier, and a staff acted out his/her erotic impulses with a patient it would be rather difficult to terminate the staff member outright without encountering legal hassles. This is especially so if the staff member says he/she was motivated "therapeutically to help the patient with his/her sexual conflicts." Granted that the behavior might be patently reprehensible, shrewd lawyers are quite adept at finding technical loopholes to shift blame elsewhere. It would be difficult indeed to argue terminating an employee on the spot if no provisions were made for informing, orienting, supervising—in short, preventing ECRs from being acted out. More telling of course, is the liability that would come from the charges of the patients's parents (or the patient himself/herself): they usually blame staff's acting out to lack of prudent administrative and clinical provisions to prevent such incidents since the institution is almost always the "deep pocket." The point being made here is *not* about whether to terminate or not to terminate staff who acted out their ECRs. The point is that it will be *very costly* to terminate staff for ECR reasons if there are no demonstrable administrative or clinical mechanisms designed to show attempts to prevent these from being acted out.

DISCUSSION

By saying that there is a need for addressing ECRs more systematically, there is the immediate danger that this will initially create a "backlash" of negative staff reactions which would be the opposite of creating a "nurturing attitude" mentioned elsewhere. This was alluded to earlier, and is analogous to the dilemma faced by well-meaning step-parents, grandparents, uncles, aunts, etc., who now feel rather self-conscious every time they give their step-children, grandchildren, nephews, or nieces a kiss, a hug, ask them to sit on their laps, give them a bath, etc. This is due to all the publicity surrounding sexual molestation of children adolescents. The same dilemma is also happening with "sexual harassment" issues in the work place although the context is somewhat different.

Where are the lines drawn? By calling attention to it, does one run the risk of getting the "innocent majority" to become defensive, less demonstrative, less spontaneous, and distant and sterile in the interactions with the patients? There are no easy answers, of course, nor pat formulas that can be offered at this time beyond the suggestions mentioned earlier of confronting the issue consciously, and of creating a "nurturing attitude," that will allow for safe identification, and therapeutic resolution. I think that any premature attempt to "quantify" what kisses are "acceptable," what parts of the body can be "therapeutically touched," what dress codes are "seductive," etc., is not only missing the point, but may well become the "problem" itself, since it could foster a "police state" mentality. And yet, having said that, there is of course a pressing need to draw lines. Child caring institutions must use administrative diligence in screening out staff who have, or are having, problems with sexual issues. There must be some explicit guidelines as to what parts of the body must *not* be touched regardless of the context. There must be explicit dress codes that clearly state what is or is not acceptable. There must be a clear statement as to which affiliative actions are not allowed.

Perhaps it is in the nature of confronting a sensitive issue that there are a lot of ambivalence and paradoxes initially. Hopefully, these ambiguities will serve as a catalyst for future studies. In the final analysis, the over-all gestalt (i.e., the "nurturing attitude") *is* the line that is drawn, and it is the over-all message, *not* the preoccupation with rules and regulations, that will lead to effective integration of ECT reactions in day to day program operations.

CONCLUSIONS

Increased awareness and sensitivity of the community to the possibility of sexual abuse of children and youth by institutional staff that were supposed to take care and treat them, has made it necessary for treatment centers to pay closer attention to the clinical and administrative implications of ECRs. Sensationalistic public reporting of alleged sexual molestations of youngsters by teachers, priests, scout leaders, child care workers, foster-parents, etc., are the more obvious and lurid manifestations of ECRs that are "acted out" by "professional staff." Not as attention-grabbing, but equally problematic, are behaviors by staff that could be construed as erotic, though not blatantly sexual. This paper has attempted to define, clarify, and explore the clinical and administrative implications of ECRs. Since it was the main contention of the paper that staff *cannot not* have ECRs when working with children and youth, the thrust of the presentation was on how to effectively integrate this naturally occurring phenomena so that it becomes not only manageable, but therapeutic.

REFERENCES

Beitman, B. Categories of Countertransference. *Journal of Operational Psychiatry*, 14(2): 82-90, 1982.

Book, H. et al. Staff Countertransference to Borderline Patients on an In-patient Unit. *American Journal of Psychotherapy*, 32(4): 521-532, 1978.

Cohen, M. Countertransference and Anxiety. *Psychiatry*, 15: 231-243, 1952.

Freud, S. The Future Prospects of Psychoanalytic Therapy. Standard Edition. London. Hogarth Press 11: 139-152, 1957.

Gartner, A. Countertransference Issues in the Psychotherapy of Adolescents. *Journal of Child and Adolescent Psychotherapy*, 2(3): 187-196, 1985.

Marcus, I. Countertransference and the Psychoanalytic Process in Children and Adolescents. Psychoanalytic Study of the Child. New Haven, CT. Yale University Press 35: 285-298, 1980.

Marshall, R. Countertransference with Children and Adolescents in Countertransference. Epstein L. and Feiner A. (Eds.) New York. Aronson, 1979.

Perkins, M. et al. Common Countertransference Issues Related to In-patient/Residential Psychiatric Treatment of Children. *The Psychiatric Hospital* 15(2): 65-74, 1984.

Realmuto, G. et al. The Management of Sexual Issues in Adolescent Treatment Programs. *Adolescence*, 21(82): 347-356, 1986.

Sandler, V. et al. Basic Psychoanalytic Concepts. IV. Countertransference. *British Journal of Psychiatry*, 117: 83-88, 1970.

Schneider, S. et al. Adolescent Sexuality in a Therapeutic Community: Staff Countertransference Issues. *Adolescence*, 20(78): 369-376, 1985.

Simpkinson, A. The Elephant in the Meditation Hall. *Common Boundary*, 8(3): 5, 1980.

Time Magazine. Six Years of Trial by Torture. January 29: 26-29, 1990.

U.S. News and World Report. The Child Abuse Trial That Left a National Legacy. January 29: 8, 1990.

Index

Administration. *See* Agency policies

Adolescents. *See* Children and adolescents

Agency policies
    adolescent sexual problems, 32
    allegations of sexual abuse by staff, 19,99-105
    erotic countertransference issues, 117-120
    hiring, 19-20
    participatory sex play, 28
    sexual behavior of clients, 35-36
    sexually stimulating media, 52-53
    support of staff, 17-19
    treatment philosophy, 116

Aggression
    exhibitionism and, 30-31
    sexually stimulating material in, 41-42,44-47

Aggressive style in survivors of sexual abuse, 82

American Psychiatric Association, 63,67

Analytic alliance, 115-116

Anderson, S.C., 66

Anger
    sexually stimulating material and, 45
    in survivors of sexual abuse, 78-79

Anne (case study), 4

Appearance and gender identity, 5-6

Armsworth, M. W., 18

Arousal reactions
    sexually stimulating material and, 43
    in survivors of sexual abuse, 83-84

The Arts in treatment, 71,79-83

Assessment in treatment of adolescent sexual offenders, 60

Attitudinal changes and sexually stimulating material, 44,46, 48,49-50

Attorney General's Commission on Pornography: Final Report, 38,44-52

Aural sexually stimulating material, 51-52

Avoider/Denier, 76-77

Bagley, C., 12,14,16,67

Barbara (case study), 6

Bauer, S. K., 67,71

Bean, G. J., 18

Beitman, B., 117

Bender, L., 67

Benign exploitation, 110-111

Berkowitz, L., 45

Berliner, L., 67

Biaggio, M. K., 67

Blau, A., 67

Bloom, Robert B., 18,19,89

Body image in survivors of sexual abuse, 80,82

Book, H., 117

Breathing exercises, 83

Briere, J., 15

Browne, A., 12,13,66

Bryant, J., 44

Burdsal, C., 58

Burgess, A. W., 67,68,83

Burnett, Richard, 57

Desensitization theory, 47
Devereux Foundation's Gateway Villas
    Treatment Programs, 66
Diane (case study), 69
Donnerstein, Edward, 38,42,43,45,
    46-47,48,50,51
Doyle, J. S., 67,71
Dress
    in gender identity, 5-6
    staff, 34
Durkin, R., 19, 91
Dynamics of sexual abuse, 10-13,68

Education in treatment, 70
Edward (case study), 28-29
Emery, P., 67,70,71
Emma (case study), 3
Emotions
    and sexually stimulating material
        in aggression, 44,49
    of staff in reaction to sexual
        abuse, 10-16
    in survivors of sexual abuse,
        12-13,69,78-79
Ernst, E., 67
Erotic countertransference issues,
    107-122
    administrative implications, 117-120
    clinical implications, 114-117
    patient-induced, 113-114
    staff-induced, 110-113
    terminology, 107-110
Executive staff, 100
Exhibitionism in childhood, 28-31

Families. *See* Parents
Family therapy for adolescent sexual
    offenders, 60
Feelings. *See* Emotions
Females
    depiction in violently sexual
        material, 45-46,49
    response to sexually stimulating
        material, 44

Feminists' view of pornography,
    41-42
Films in aggression, 46,50
Finkelhor, D., 66
First Amendment, 39-40
Fisher, S., 80
Flossie (case study), 6
Force, R., 58
Fraser Committee, 42
Freud, S., 108

Gender identity
    medical problems and, 33
    physical appearance and, 5-6
Genitourinary problems, 33
Giarretto, H., 10
Gil, E., 67
Gillman, R., 15
Girls. *See also* Children and
        adolescents
    physical affection with men, 1-8
    physical appearance and gender
        identity, 5-6
Goodill, S. W., 81,82
Grace (case study), 4
Groth, N., 67
Group therapy. *See also* Treatment
    for adolescent sexual offenders,
        59
    for survivors of sexual abuse,
        71,73,75-84
Groze, V., 18
Grugett, A. E., 67

Haaken, J., 14
Hartman, C. R., 67,68
Herman, J. L., 13,14,17
Heterogeneous milieu in treatment of
        adolescent sexual
        offenders, 62-63
Hicho, D., 18
Hiring policies, 19-20
Holstrom, L., 67
Home visits